Conquering Yeast Infections
The Non-Drug Solution for Men and Women

Conquering

Yeast

Infections

THE NON-DRUG SOLUTION
FOR MEN AND WOMEN

S. Colet Lahoz, RN, MS, LAc

Pentland Press, Inc.
ENGLAND ● USA ● SCOTLAND

PUBLISHED BY PENTLAND PRESS, INC.
5124 Bur Oak Circle, Raleigh, North Carolina 27612
United States of America
919-782-0281

ISBN 1-57197-016-9
Library of Congress Catalog Card Number 96-67040

Printed in the United States of America

This book is dedicated to my husband, Tom and my son Mark Jensen for their loving presence in my life.

Special thanks to Monica O'Kane, Dr. Thomas Fiutak, Lauri Ross O'Kane, and Lucena Deniega for their help in the editing and research process.

To all my patients who participated in the study, specially to Sharon Scully, Terry Bateman, Dr. Kevin Keough, Anne and Mary Bajari who taught me a lot about the treatment of CRC.

About the Author

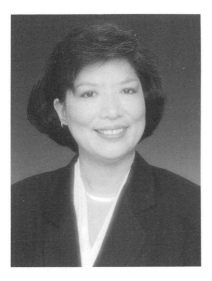

Colet Lahoz, a licensed acupuncturist in Minnesota has operated her own holistic clinic, the East West Clinic, since 1984. After receiving her bachelor of nursing degree from St. Paul College in Manila, Philippines (1965) she continued her career in the United States. Upon completing her masters degree in nursing from the University of Minnesota she returned to the Philippines in 1981 to pursue a postgraduate course in traditional Chinese medicine.

Her career as a registered nurse included staff positions in critical care and trauma, pioneering the development of emergency and trauma courses for nurses. She held faculty positions at the Beth Israel School of Nursing in New York City, where she taught advanced neurology, and the University of Minnesota in Minneapolis. She was director of nursing education at Children's Hospital in St. Paul, Minnesota.

Table of Contents

Foreword

It has been nearly two decades since C. Orian Truss, M.D., an allergist in Birmingham, Alabama presented to a medical forum his observation that depressed patients are affected by a yeast organism, called Candida albicans. This yeast was not a new or unique discovery as it had been treated by gynecologists and pediatricians for years in the form of vaginitis in women and thrush in infants. What was remarkable about Truss's report was drawing the relationship between clinical depression, a "mental" disorder, and yeast, an infective organism usually associated only with superficial human infections. Truss presented a series of papers on the injury the yeast organism, Candida, subjects to the human body in the *Journal of Orthomolecular Medicine*. By the early 1980s, other physicians interested in chronic illness and allergy began to explore yeast's relationship in causing numerous unexplained illnesses. This led to Dr. Billy Crook publishing *The Yeast Connection* in 1984 as well as Drs. John Trowbridge and Morton Walker writing *The Yeast Syndrome* in 1986. By the late 1980s the medical community became divided into two camps: those who "believed" in the condition known as systemic candidiasis or CRC and those who did not believe in it. The believers largely consisted of alternative medical practitioners who already subscribed to many theories lying outside the medical mainstream; the non-believers began to publish editorials in the orthodox medical journals claiming that the yeast syndrome was a fad and did not have any legitimacy in medical diagnosis or treatment.

While this disconcerting set of events has made candidiasis a difficult condition to work with both as a patient and as a physician, there have been many rewards for both in pursuing understanding the yeast syndrome. Chronic illness frequently is diagnosed in very black-and-white terms, such as arthritis, asthma, ulcer, and psoriasis. However, many chronic conditions are undiagnosed and present incredible frustration for doctor and patient. For example, many patients have at a relatively young age, 30-40, difficulties with remembering and calculating simple sales register receipts. Obviously, it is very unlikely that these individuals have major brain disorders such as Alzheimer's. But what can explain these lessened abilities to think in apparently normal persons? Others continue to experience recurrent upper respiratory infections, sinusitis, sore throats, ear infections, and colds with no apparent cause. Despite numerous rounds of antibiotics, even throat or ear surgery, they continue to have infection after infection. Other patients yet have terrible digestive tract disorders with continuous gas, indigestion, diarrhea, constipation, bloating and heartburn trying all sorts of medications and diets with little relief of their symptoms. What could be the cause of these symptoms? As unbelievable as it may be to many patients and doctors, this often ignored yeast, Candida, can frequently be the culprit. Yet, Candida can not just be "eliminated." We all look for the simple pill to cure all our problems; candida is just not responsive to the magic bullet.

We know that there is a relationship between Candida and these chronic illnesses because when we treat the yeast and have the patient follow programs designed to control the yeast, the patient responds remarkably, even after many previous medical treatment programs for unrelated conditions failed. Even the patient who previously failed with "quick" anti-yeast treatment, will respond if a program is designed with an appropriate anti-yeast diet, long-term use of anti-candida supplements and/or medications, complementary nutritional supplementation including herbals, vitamins, minerals, amino acids, whole food supplements, and homeopathic supports. In addition, other modalities, such as acupuncture, traditional Chinese medicine, and naturopathy play an important role in supporting the restoration of the candida patient to their normal condition.

It has been quite difficult to develop research studies on treating patients having chronic illness, labeled candidiasis or CRC, when candida may not be quickly diagnosed by a standardized test. Further, even when the patient and physician are open to treating candida, the usual quick one or two course treatments of anti-yeast Nystatin or Nizoral or Diflucan are usually insufficient to eradicate the more chronic illness. S. Colet Lahoz, RN, a nurse and acupuncturist in Minnesota, decided to undertake a research study of diagnosing and treating candidiasis employing a well-scheduled program of diet, anti-candida fungicide, nutritional supportive supplements as well as acupuncture. The study followed patients who scored high on questionnaires designed to screen for candidiasis reported by Crook and Trowbridge. Patients were asked to compare their symptom responses following essentially no anti-yeast program, a medication program, or the program designed by Lahoz involving diet, a four part anti-candida colon cleansing program, as well as nutritional supplementation. The results of the study demonstrated candida symptoms could be very well controlled by patients who followed a rigorous dietary and colon cleansing program compared to patients who only followed diet and anti-candida medication. More remarkable for those patients was the constancy of symptom response for those who completed the bowel cleansing program. The study strongly suggests that the yeast syndrome is not only tied into many of these chronic illnesses, but that the bowel or digestive system is the primary site where yeast settle in the body and produce the toxic by-products which bring on the vast array of symptoms throughout the body. It argues again for the theory the hygienists championed a century earlier: that an unhealthy lower bowel is the breeding ground for infection and inflammation which will cause illness throughout the body. That cleaning out the lower bowel will only improve an individuals health; ignoring the bowel's hygiene will lead to more generalized chronic illness.

Conquering Yeast Infections, The Non-Drug Solution by S. Colet Lahoz, RN, LAc is a book for believers in the yeast syndrome as well as patients and physicians who have been frustrated by difficulties in managing candidiasis. It describes in a very readable format the basis for candida as cause of chronic illness as well as the theory behind its causation. Lahoz reviews the difficulty in diagnosing candida by conventional laboratory testing and examines the tools most practitioners who diagnose and treat CRC use in evaluating new and long-standing patients. She presents the data Drs. Truss, Crook, Trowbridge and

Walker, and others have published on diagnosing and treating yeast syndrome. Lahoz presents the components of her four-part colon cleansing program, including an anti-candidal oil called Caprol, as well as a clay cleanser, bentonite, a well-known fiber support, psyllium and the implantation of friendly, colon organisms, acidophilus. The colon cleansing program is used twice daily with the anti-candida diet for a period of three months to effectively clean the colon of yeast organism and yeast toxins. Following the theory, Lahoz presents data following candida patients who actively followed the yeast program. Lahoz also provides guidelines for managing life following the completion of the yeast treatment. Throughout the text patient profiles are presented which clearly reveal the difficulties many patients of all ages have experienced in diagnosing their chronic illness, obtaining effective help for their condition, and the change in their life once the candida was effectively controlled. Except for minor irritable periods when the yeast "die off," the program Lahoz proposes poses few significant side effects.

We have all spent considerable energies looking to find answers to long-term chronic complaints, often with no better advice than our symptoms represent psychological stress. Lahoz's *Conquering Yeast Infections* tells a different story, one that most assuredly affects millions of Americans, who never receive any relief until their condition turns from symptom and illness to major disease. Why do we need to wait for major disease before we get help? Why not consider the cause before our body degenerates and threatens critical illness? I would highly recommend that *Conquering Yeast Infections* be required reading for doctors and patients who are getting nowhere treating long-standing unsolved illness.

—Jonathan Collin, MD
Editor-in-Chief, *Townsend Letter for Doctors and Patients*
May 1996

Introduction

I decided to write about yeast infections for several reasons. As a nurse I have watched with concern the professional controversy surrounding this illness. Because of this controversy, or possibly because of an unawareness of it, many physicians do not diagnose and treat Candida Related Complex (CRC).

Consequently, the alternative professions of naturopathy, chiropractic, acupuncture, and herbal medicine have dealt with these cases and have contributed a great deal to the understanding of this illness. I met many people—men, women, and even children as young as infants—affected with this very complex problem. My heart went out to these sick patients as they struggled with their misery. I listened to their stories and witnessed them go from doctor to doctor seeking help for their various symptoms.

Then I met a special person at a conference for holistic practitioners. She was intrigued by my work in acupuncture and wanted to know if it could help her particular problems. This serendipitous connection resulted in many life-changing events affecting both of our lives. I learned that she had suffered from CRC for over 35 years, and was often severely debilitated by it until she found the right combination of products to treat her problems. She told me that knowledge of these products was the answer to her prayers for a healthy recovery. Her story appears in Case Study Six of this book. In short, how she used this program to get well produced the answer that I had been searching for. Her story gave me the incentive to start a study using this program along with acupuncture and diet for CRC patients.

This book is about the study of approximately sixty people for a period of two years. They are the stories of men, women, and children who are now fully recovered from CRC. They share stories about which combination of treatments worked, which ones were least beneficial, the importance of adhering to a healthy diet, and the overwhelmingly positive results of this program, acupuncture, and other therapies. An estimated 79 million Americans have this disease today and only a very small percentage are accurately diagnosed. Still fewer are in a treatment program that gives them long-term relief.

—S. Colet Lahoz, RN, MS, LAc

Part One
Candida Related Complex

Case Study One

39-Year-Old-Female Diagnosed with Cardiomyopathy

"You need a heart transplant, Sharon Scully," was the strong pronouncement from Dr. Cheng, the cardiologist who evaluated my echocardiogram on 24 May 1993. Immediately, I realized what a major decision I had to make, despite the fact that I was only thirty-nine years old. The thought was very depressing.

For the last fourteen years I had been searching for a drug-free way to deal with chronic asthma that I have had since childhood. I was finally beginning to understand the value of nutrition and supplements. I was able to break the cycle of drugs, prednisone, and antibiotics for the treatment of recurrent asthmatic episodes and infections common to asthmatics like myself. My husband Richard and I worked as a team to regain control of my life and my illness. We learned about food combining, the hazards of sugar, and the benefits of healthy eating. My system was finally detoxifying after years of prescription drug use. A year into this new lifestyle, I became pregnant and was fortunate enough to find midwives who helped me deliver at home.

My health was getting better, except for recurrent and persistent skin itching and irritation that the doctors could not treat. When we moved to Minnesota in 1985, I had been free of drugs for five years. Then I had another severe episode of asthma and decided to try acupuncture. I was fortunate to meet Colet, an acupuncture therapist in 1986 who has been helping me keep my asthma under control since then. She is truly gifted. She would get me balanced and off I'd go for weeks or months until I needed another tune up. She also introduced me to the supplement called KM by Matol. She said it was the cell food I needed to get my body detoxified and better nourished. The effects were astonishing. I had more energy and the ability to bounce back more quickly when I became sick.

Looking back at the months leading to my heart failure, I recall that there was a lot of stress. Among other things, we had moved to the country and gotten a large mortgage. I was just starting to build my own distributorship with KM. Earlier in May of 1993, my asthma took a turn for the worse again. My inhalers did not seem to work anymore, and my feet and hands had swollen. I had insomnia, felt a lot of nausea, and could not tolerate any food intake. I tried to schedule a doctor's appointment but they were booked up. No one could see me right away. I rapidly gained weight—twelve pounds in fourteen days.

Finally, I went to urgent care. The doctor's diagnosis was "walking pneumonia" and he prescribed antibiotics and cortisone. I asked about the sudden weight gain and he said that I looked like I was just fat and sent me home. The prescription drugs made my condition worse. Now it felt like my internal organs were all under pressure and were about to burst. So, I returned to the hospital. This time they were concerned about kidney failure and put me on massive doses of diuretics. An echocardiogram showed severe congestive heart failure, which was unusual for my age.

A series of consultations, including a heart biopsy, failed to reveal the cause. They could not find any reason for the congestive heart failure and the subsequent cardiomyopathy. It was a mystery. The doctor said I should get my name on the transplant list for heart donors because it was my only hope. They wanted me to start a regimen of steroids to prepare my body for the transplant. They found the story of my lifelong quest to be drug-free very humorous under the circumstances.

Nine days later, I left the hospital determined to find an alternative to a heart transplant. I made two phone calls as soon as I got home. One to my friend Reed D. Bolander, who has been my resource for herbal and nutrient information. He recommended that I start taking red cayenne pepper right away.

The second phone call was to the acupuncture therapist. She started seeing me three times a week. She said my pulses showed a severe deficiency of yang elements and of chi (the energy of life that is assessed by palpating the pulses in the radial artery on both wrists). My heart and small intestine pulses, which represent the fire element, were almost totally nonpalpable. The only way she could tell I had a heart beat was by listening to my heart with a stethoscope. No wonder I was so fatigued. I no longer could take walks. Climbing a flight of stairs was almost impossible. The acupuncture therapist suggested that I take Coenzyme Q-10 to improve my heart's capacity to pump. She used a combination of acupuncture and moxibustion to stimulate more chi in my energy channels.

After two months on this regimen, I was somewhat better but nothing significant was happening. I also began to have increased itching; even my ears and eyes were itching. This gave the acupuncture therapist the clue that, because of my repeated use of antibiotics and prednisone in the past, I may have developed systemic candidiasis. The Candida questionnaire showed a definite yes. I had an overwhelming fungus infection. She felt that this may be the answer to the mystery surrounding my heart failure. She said that once the fungus overgrows the body, it can invade any organ, even the heart, as in my case. She then suggested that I take the fungicide and colon cleanser herbal mix (Acu-Trol brand) and go on a yeast-free, sugar-free diet. I also continued acupuncture twice a week.

The next few weeks were miraculous. My heart finally pumped more efficiently, my skin cleared up, and my eyes and ears no longer itched. My progress from that point was rapid. I was able to take walks again for twenty to forty minutes at a time. I was able to slowly increase my endurance by using the rebounder (a miniature trampoline). My improvement confirmed our hunch that the Candida had invaded my heart muscles and caused the heart failure. Now, because I was cleaning the fungus out of my body, it was only a matter of time before I recovered. The acupuncture treatments were needed to restore my heart function, as well as the function of the rest of my organs, which had gone through a major shutdown. It seems that the recurrent pulmonary episodes in the past were also Candida-related because now that I am in treatment, my lungs are better than ever. My therapist also introduced me to some herbal anti-asthmatic pills. Some are Chinese formulations and some are Western herbs. They have been very effective in controlling my asthma.

I continued on the regimen of acupuncture, fungicides, herbal colon cleansers, and a strict diet for ten months. I have now reached my one-year anniversary after the diagnosis of cardiomyopathy. My doctor finally agreed that I was in good health. All my tests showed that my heart was improved. Furthermore, none of my other organs were showing signs of failure. My doctor was very surprised and said, "I don't understand what the others are doing for you, but whatever it is, it must be good because you are indeed better." My parents were the ones who most needed to hear this from the doctor, because the entire time I was going to the therapist, they had worried that I was doing the wrong thing. They feared that I was going to die.

In May of 1994, I celebrated my fortieth birthday—a true celebration of life. This birthday was also a thanksgiving for the wonderful healer who has found a drug-free, non-surgical way to help people like myself.

—Sharon Scully, Annandale, Minnesota

Chapter One

The Definition of Candida Related Complex

Candida albicans is the specific name for a strain of a normally peaceful, yeast-like fungus naturally existing in limited amounts in our digestive tract from our mouth to our rectum—especially in dark, moist places. It is a harmless parasite which is carried by a significant percentage of people. It is a plant, although it behaves like an animal; it uses oxygen, has an animal-like nucleus in each cell, and has a metabolism similar to an animal.

In healthy individuals, Candida albicans occurs in small colonies and coexists with beneficial microbes or bacteria. The presence of yeast and bacteria in controlled balance does not cause any problems.

Yeast, in its many varieties, is a unicellular fungus that reproduces by budding spores. It looks like a foam or froth and is capable of fermenting carbohydrates. As a fungus, yeast contains enzymes that can digest material from humans.

Besides Candida albicans, another fungus that most people are familiar with is a mold sometimes found on old bread and cheese. Mold is caused by fungus which in turn causes disintegration of organic matter. Whether it is Candida albicans or any of its related species, fungus causes a weakening of the cellular structure in which it lives. This explains why patients afflicted with this type of infection become very ill and are difficult to treat; many of their cells become weak. People who have tried to remove mold in their walls or basement rugs can attest to the difficulty in eliminating this type of infestation. Fungus is tenacious.

Many times this fungal overgrowth occurs only in localized parts of our bodies. However, these conditions can become chronic. Examples are: athlete's foot, thrush, vaginitis, or urethral candidiasis in males.

Various fungi are attracted to specific parts of humans. Thus, Candida albicans gravitates to the gastrointestinal tract, Aspergillus to the respiratory tract, Trichophyton to the feet, and Monilia to the vagina.

For instance, every year 12 million American women suffer from vaginitis—a yeast infection in the vagina. This in turn prompts approximately 22 million doctor visits annually. At some time in their lives, 75% of all women will experience vaginitis. Vaginitis is so common and the symptoms are so clear-cut, that the

Food and Drug Administration (FDA), in a December 3, 1990 press release, changed the status of the drug commonly prescribed for vaginitis, clotrimazole, to an over-the-counter (OTC) treatment.[1] This OTC product is now called Gyne-Lotrimin.

Localized fungal overgrowth, such as the above-mentioned vaginitis, are easily treated when they are the only site of the fungal infection.

Conversely, Candida Related Complex (CRC) is certainly not easily treated. It occurs when the living yeast gains entrance to the bloodstream and the lymphatics. Their mode of entrance is two-fold.

The first is by way of penetration of their root-like tentacles into the intestinal wall. This penetration destroys the mucous membrane system of the intestines. Some people call this leaking of toxins into the bloodstream the "leaky gut syndrome."

The second is by passing through the intestinal wall. This was documented in a study which proved that Candida albicans can escape the gut and travel into the bloodstream and urine in just a few hours. One dedicated, fearless researcher ingested 80 g. Candida albicans in order to investigate the fate of orally administered Candida albicans. Fungus cells were cultured from blood samples taken after three and six hours, and from urine samples after two and three hours. The blood and urine test was negative for Candida albicans. This experiment proved that Candida albicans could have entered the circulating blood only by persorption through the intestinal wall.[2]

If CRC is uncontrolled, it can cause new symptoms throughout the body and aggravate existing conditions. CRC can produce a weakening of the entire system and a lowering of resistance to other diseases.

CRC is the most dreaded complication of fungal infections, because it is very hard to recognize and even harder to treat. This differs from localized infections in that the fungi overgrowth predominates in the gastrointestinal tract, especially in the colon, and from there can penetrate other organs and systems.

Ultimately, CRC is capable of causing serious disease and even death. The balance between bacteria normally in the gut and/or vaginal flora and fungus is disrupted when the bacteria become weakened and the fungi become too strong. As a result of this imbalance, the Candida albicans can rapidly multiply and cause an overgrowth.

In CRC, one of the first systems to be compromised is the immune system. It forces the immune system to focus on the digestive tract, the source of CRC. As the immune system becomes overburdened, physical problems (caused by the rampant spread of Candida albicans through the bloodstream) proliferate. Thus, people with chronic lung problems such as asthma and bronchitis easily develop Candida pneumonia as a complication. Premenstrual syndrome (PMS) becomes even worse in women with candidiasis. In other words, any weak system becomes even weaker and more compromised after CRC. The result is a persistent condition that does not improve with conventional therapies and often gets worse following drug therapy.

This spread of Candida albicans has been described as a domino effect—one body system after another falls prey to CRC, unless it is stopped or reversed.

Pathologists studying disseminated candidiasis find tiny abscesses through-out the body. These consist of Candida albicans surrounded by a fibrin (a protein able to clot) and a connective tissue shell. This shell isolates Candida from elimination by the immune system.

Another name for CRC is "mycotoxins." This word is derived from the Greek words "myukes," meaning fungus, and "toxicum," meaning toxin or poison. "Mycotoxin is the generic term used to describe a fungal-produced toxic metabolic which can cause disease leading to death," says A. V. Constantini, M.D., head of World Health Organization (WHO) Collaborating Center for Mycotoxins in Food.

CRC is also known as Candida, candidiasis, candidiasis hypersensitivity, systemic candidiasis, CASO (Candida Albicans Systemic Overgrowth), mold, fungus, or intestinal yeast infection.

Metabolism is the process by which carbohydrates, proteins, fats, and other ingested food substances are converted into essential material for the composition of cells. If toxins are present, then the cells are being nourished with poiso-

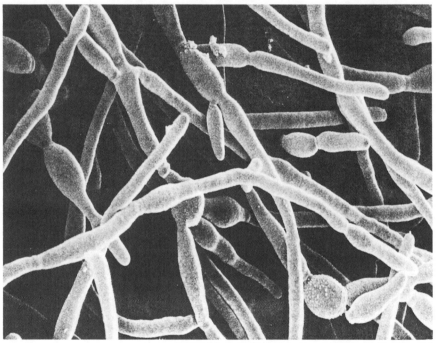

Reprinted, By Permission of the New England Journal of Medicine. (Vol. 328, 1993, p. 1322)
A scanning electron micrograph shows a pure culture of Candida albicans (x6030).

nous or toxic substances. Understandably, this process does not make for healthy cells. "The modes of entry are ingestion, inhalation, or skin contact . . . Mycotoxins in human health is a new field in medicine," says Dr. Constantini; "It brings to the scientific world, particularly the medical community, a new etiologic (cause or origin) concept which implicates the toxicogenic fungi and their specific toxins (mycotoxins) as the cause of major non-communicable disease." [3]

Orian Truss, M.D., a pioneer in the work with CRC, says that this disease causes the formation of a toxin called acetaldehyde which effects multi-system abnormalities. Acetaldehyde, a volatile, pungent gaseous compound "produced in the intestine by the fermentation of sugars (or digestible carbohydrates) by Candida albicans, is the principal mediator of metabolic disturbances." Dr. Truss' hypothesis is that acetaldehyde is the major toxin responsible for abnormalities found in CRC patients. Those with acetaldehyde poisoning exhibit significant toxic effects of excess gas, such as abdominal distention, flatulence, and belching. "The ultimate effect of this very toxic substance," Dr. Truss writes, "could include disruption of intestinal absorptive processes." [4]

Disrupting the intestinal absorptive processes results in two widely differing physical characteristics in those infected with CRC. These patients can become extremely thin because their food passes too quickly through their gastrointestinal tract. Other patients can become overweight, some even obese. In these individuals, no matter how much food they eat, their nutritional needs are not met; therefore they are often hungry within an hour or two of eating.

The mucous membranes in healthy people have a coating of mucous and immunoglobulin that helps fight fungi. Immunologist Patricia Lucas, Ph.D., has hypothesized that the major causes of immune disorders are defects in the gastrointestinal mucosa due to Candida. Lucas presented scientific data to the Society for Clinical Ecology supporting her hypotheses that Candida causes multiple hypersensitivities by first damaging the lining of the gastrointestinal tract.

Chapter Two

The Cause of Candida Related Complex

An important question is what causes the disruption in the normal balance of fungi and bacteria resulting in CRC. These causes of disruptions fall into the following categories:

1. Drug therapy, particularly antibiotics and corticosteroids (immunosuppressant type of drugs);
2. Diet high in sugar, breads, alcoholic beverages, and other food items with yeast as an ingredient;
3. Oral contraceptive hormones;
4. Stress and exhaustion; and
5. Mold in environment.

CRC is a side effect of modern medicine. Since 1950 "the increasing use of antibiotics, contraceptive hormones, and immunosuppressant drugs in medical practice has encouraged the growth of this yeast in many individuals."[1] These drugs disrupt the flora balance in the intestines.

A history of repeated use of antibiotics or prednisone or both (even as early as childhood) is one of the main causes of CRC. This can happen after prolonged (several months or more) or repeated (more than three times in 12 months) treatments with antibiotics. When bacteria are destroyed by antibiotics, the fungi grow. In essence, one infection is traded for another.

Disease that impairs the immune system makes it susceptible to CRC. When an illness places a burden on the immune system and the patient is given immunosuppressant drugs, the body cannot fight the spread of fungi and they multiply.

The development of Candida albicans from a harmless fungus to a common cause of hospital-acquired infectious disease is frightening. The medical community has pursued advanced technology for sustaining life, including organ transplants, artificial joints, long-term dialysis, and chemotherapy. The techniques used in these new technologies enable Candida albicans to invade deep organs. [2]

The severity of hospital-acquired infections merited the formation of the National Nosocomial (hospital-acquired) Infections Surveillance System. During the 1980s, this group reported studying 344,610 nosocomial pathogens (disease-producing microorganisms). They discovered that 7.9% were fungi and the Candida species accounted for 79% of these fungi. "Unfortunately, a disturbingly large number of patients die with undiagnosed invasive Candida infections," reports an editorial in the *New England Journal of Medicine*. This editorial also states that the mortality rate is from 38 to 59% of patients with candidemia (Candida in the blood). "Our advanced technology for sustained life support is predominantly responsible for creating the current relation of the organisms with the human host." [3]

A study reported at the 1988 CRC Update compared five Candida diets. At the top of each list was a restriction against consumption of refined sugar. This food item feeds the fungi allowing them to proliferate; it is addictive and overconsumption is the norm; it causes an imbalance in acid/alkaline levels, wreaks havoc with the sugar/insulin blood ratio (causing physical stress), and increases the physical need for vitamins and minerals. [4]

Many people don't realize the hidden sugar content in foods and beverages. There are seven teaspoons of sugar in each can of soda, a similar amount of sugar in each shot of liquor, and many "salty" foods such as catsup are also high in sugar.

Because of poor dietary habits, "junk food" eaters are at high risk of developing this condition. Candida albicans feeds on sugar and foods baked with yeast. People with CRC develop a craving for sweets, often describing an insatiable urge to eat sugar or bread or drink beer or other alcoholic beverages. Many sufferers attribute this to poor self control and often have shame and guilt associated with this craving and binging. What many do not realize is that their cravings are caused by the yeast they are harboring which is begging to be fed.

Another dietary factor is the regular consumption of poultry, meat, and milk. The animals from which we get these products have been treated with antibiotics and hormones that are then passed on to the consumer of the meat or milk, thus destroying good bacteria in the gut of the consumer. Chemical preservatives present in many foods also encourage CRC.

Low bulk, highly-refined carbohydrate diets also help establish a breeding ground for yeast. This diet slows the peristaltic action of the colon (the washing machine-like movement of the colon). A sluggish colon builds up layers of fecal matter in the large intestine. This layering results in putrefaction, fermentation and rancidification of old ingested food, which is a perfect home for Candida albicans. On this diet, the small intestine becomes clogged with mucous which promotes the growth of fungus.

Adult women are afflicted with CRC much more frequently than other groups. Sixty percent of the CRC patients are women, 20% men, and 20% children. Babies, as they descend through the birth canal, can be exposed to Candida, often developing a fungal mouth thrush and fungal diaper rash soon after birth.

In women, the fluctuation of hormones tends to predispose them to a weaker immune system and lessened resistance to CRC. Additionally, the female anatomy—with the vagina in close proximity to the rectum—lends itself to easy migration of Candida albicans.

Oral contraceptives contain synthetic progesterone which change the lining of the vagina, making it easier for women to develop CRC. This overgrowth can then easily spread to the intestines.

Stress and exhaustion can predispose one to CRC by placing an enormous burden on the immune system. Stress of illness or overwork and/or trauma from the loss of a loved one or a job is often a causative agent of CRC.

Fungi in our environment can bring on an exaggeration of CRC symptoms. Fungi grows both inside and outside our homes. It likes dark, damp places like basements, sinks, rugs, closets, old magazines or newspapers, flowerpots, stored fresh foods, shady areas in the yard, and piles of dead leaves. Tobacco is manufactured by application of a great deal of sugar (in the curing mixture) to the leaves, and this curing process allows various yeast and fungi to grow.

Additionally, firewood often contains fungi. Usually trees are cut after the tree has sprouted fungi. When this contaminated wood is burned in a fireplace, many Candida patients will react to the smoke.

Actually, there are two types of CRC. The first is intestinal and is mainly a result of the food we eat. The second is respiratory and is produced by contact with the pollen of weeds, grasses and trees, house dust, and animal dander. Thus, CRC is caused by either diet or environment.

Chapter Three

Assessment and Analysis of Symptoms

Identifying and diagnosing Candida Related Complex (CRC) is difficult and can easily be missed unless the health care professional is proficient in the intricacies of its symptoms.

Author and nutritional consultant Rupert Beebe states that diagnosing the CRC patient is difficult because the patient is neither sick nor well, has many complaints and health problems, yet is without sufficient definitive symptoms to make a definite diagnosis. [1]

The complexity of the manifestations of CRC is a stumbling block for many in identifying this ailment as the cause of a chronic multi-system illness. Research into a similar situation, however, demonstrates that such a wide-ranging malady is indeed possible. Joseph Goldberger, M.D. (1874-1929), proved that pellagra is caused by a vitamin B deficiency. Pellagra causes skin changes, gastrointestinal disturbances, and nervous disorders. Persons with this illness suffer from diarrhea, dermatitis, and dementia—it is a multi-system illness. With pellagra, the seemingly unrelated organs of the intestine, skin, and brain all show abnormal function. Even though they are separated from each other in the body, all share the same metabolic pathways which require adequate vitamin B3. [2] This discovery established a precedent for one illness which affects several systems. Like pellagra, CRC can have a multi-system involvement.

There are several factors that make it difficult to identify the existence of CRC.

First, the symptoms vary widely and can be manifested in many ways. Most physicians who are not specifically looking to rule out CRC as the underlying cause for particular symptoms can easily overlook its possibility. This often results in patients being treated solely for their overt problems.

The difficulty in identifying CRC leaves many physicians unconvinced and skeptical of the existence of this illness. Patients are often told that if their symptoms do not respond to prescribed treatments or if the symptoms return again shortly after treatment ceases, then the symptoms must be psychosomatic.

Second, many physicians feel that laboratory tests are not very reliable in identifying CRC. Soon after birth, all healthy individuals demonstrate the presence of the fungus Candida albicans in their intestinal tract. This is a normal occurrence. But many health care professionals believe that cultures and smears will not be able to determine if there is an overgrowth of the fungus.

A 1991 *New England Journal of Medicine* article agrees that blood cultures are uncertain.

> Diagnosing the invasion of deep organs by Candida has been problematic for two reasons. First, patients may have extensive invasive Candida infections of several deep organs, yet have negative blood cultures. Second, the meaning of a positive blood culture for Candida has been questioned, especially during the early years of the organism's emergence as a pathogen. [3]

Author John Edwards, M.D., feels that diagnosing CRC is perplexing because even though patients may have this illness, their stool culture may not always support the facts. Even if the stool cultures are positive, analysts do not always agree as to the meaning of the results.

The authors of another report in the same issue of this journal state,

> Invasive candidiasis is a major nosocomial (hospital-acquired) infection that is difficult to diagnose. Few biochemically defined markers of invasive candidiasis are known. Initial findings suggested that the presence of Candida enolase (enzyme) in the blood may be a novel marker for invasive candidiasis. [4]

The above researchers state that CRC is a major infection that some people acquire while in the hospital for a separate illness. There are not many markers in the blood to show CRC. However, new findings suggest that blood containing Candida enzymes may be a sign of CRC.

Fortunately, a study published later in the *Journal of Advancement in Medicine* reports a positive relationship between Candida albicans and baker's yeast as indicated by an enzyme radioallergosorbent test (RAST). This test measures immunoglobulin-E (IgE) reactivity of antibody immunoglobulins produced by the body and directed against Candida antigens. IgE measures the allergic response to a specific food or inhalant with symptoms appearing within six to eight hours after exposure. The RAST, which accurately measures the overgrowth of Candida albicans in the bloodstream, has been approved by the FDA.[5] Furthermore, there are other laboratory tests which can be used to determine CRC. However, many alternative health care professionals feel that these laboratory tests are not essential in diagnosis and treatment of CRC.

It has been proven that CRC can be successfully diagnosed and treated without laboratory tests. For example, fungal expert and author John Parks Trowbridge, M.D., feels that a clinical diagnosis of CRC can be based on the ratings of a self-administered questionnaire of the patient's health, their personal clinical history, a physical examination, possibly an anti-Candida antibody test, and the patient's response to a therapeutic CRC treatment program. [6]

Food addiction specialist Douglas Hunt, M.D., believes that many patients who have undiagnosed CRC will manifest unexplained, difficult-to-diagnose symptoms. One of the most prominent symptoms caused by CRC is intense cravings for sweets, breads, and cheeses. It is this symptom which he believes is a good indicator of CRC. Cravings for alcoholic beverages such as beer and wine are another clue. [7]

These cravings are frequent and intense. Many patients are convinced there is something terribly wrong with them psychologically or behaviorally and they often have greatly diminished self-esteem. There is a lot of shame and guilt associated with this phenomenon. These patients do not freely divulge this information unless asked. If a treatment program is working, these cravings will disappear.

Allergist and best-selling author William Crook, M.D., feels that a CRC diagnosis can be suspected from the patient's history, which may include the usual symptoms of the CRC person, particularly chronic fatigue. When these symptoms are present, a program is initiated including anti-fungal treatment, vitamin supplementation, diet modification (primarily eliminating refined sugar), and avoiding chemicals. Then, if the patient's health improves, the diagnosis is confirmed by the positive reaction to the treatment. [8]

Some guidelines are offered to alternative practitioners who are trying to become knowledgeable about the diagnosis and treatment of CRC. The following complaints are the signals that could indicate the possibility of CRC.

The patient experiences a combination of fatigue, mood swings, irritability, anxiety, depression, and headaches, combined with poor dietary habits, chronic stress, and little or no tolerance for exercise. These symptoms are intensified on damp and muggy days or when in moldy places such as basements.

Patients complain of abdominal bloating as a recurrent problem. They might use phrases like, "My abdomen hurts, and It gets so bad that I have to use clothes with an elastic waist or no waist because my usual clothes do not fit;" "My lower left abdomen feels stuck;" "Many times I feel all right just before my bowel movement in the morning, but soon after that I feel pain and a tightness in the lower abdomen;" or "I feel weakened and even confused." This bloating happens frequently, often several times daily. Once it starts, it takes a long time for it to go away.

There is often a link between the type of food ingested and the occurrence of this type of bloating. Foods that cause this reaction are those high in sugar and starch, and beer and wine. In severe situations almost any type of food ingested will trigger this reaction. A person in this extreme situation of reacting to most foods is called a universal food reactor. Those reacting to smells are called chemical reactors. They react to many odors including perfumes, chemicals, molds, auto exhaust, pesticides and cleaning solvents. So CRC patients can be sensitive to either food or their environment or both.

Another major clue to the presence of CRC is a history of the person having been treated with antibiotics, birth control pills, or corticosteroids. (Steroids come in the form of drugs such as Prednisone, Decadron, Prednisolone, etc.). Patients are told to ask their parents if, as young children, they were often sick with infections such as earaches, bronchitis, and strep throat. If so, they are then to ask if they were treated with repeated doses of antibiotics.

Recurrent infections (sinusitis, earaches, urinary tract infections, vaginal infections, bronchitis, etc.) that do not respond to antibiotics or prednisone therapy or keep recurring after drug treatment, is another clue. In fact, in most cases patients get worse with these drug therapies because the fungal-bacterial ratio is compromised even more. It is often at this point that patients finally seek alternative healers after experiencing no success with their allopathic doctors.

Recurrent, severe allergies that do not respond or respond minimally to anti-histamines (anti-allergy medications) is another red flag. These sensitivities include a wide range of symptoms: nasal drainage, gastrointestinal disturbances, sensitivity to scents and fumes, or skin eruptions with itching that can affect any part of the body but often occur in the armpits, groin, and under the nails. Many people are so sensitive that inhaling chemicals in ordinary cleaning sprays used in homes and offices make them weak for days.

Molds in closets, rugs, basements, and other moist places cause nasal drainage and extreme tiredness. Patients with an advanced condition showing allergy as a predominant symptom find themselves unable to go to many public places—severely limiting their lifestyle.

Identifying and diagnosing CRC is difficult because of the complexity of this multi-system illness. Most physicians who are not specifically looking for CRC can easily overlook this cause of illness. Many alternative health care professionals feel that laboratory tests are not essential. Most CRC experts feel that if this illness is strongly suspected by specific symptoms evidenced by questionnaire responses (such as cravings, chronic fatigue, abdominal bloating, and excessive antibiotic use), then an anti-fungal program and diet modifications should be instituted. Improvement in the patient's health will confirm the CRC suspicion.

Case Study Two

45-Year-Old Female with Anxiety, Palpitations, Ringing in Ears

I am a 45-year-old female, married with two grown children. I tried acupuncture therapy for the first time in February, 1994. I went to see an acupuncturist based on the recommendation of a friend who had gone to the acupuncturist for chronic health problems. I had been having heart palpitations, anxiety, and ringing in my ears, which was worse in my right ear.

I had initially consulted my physician for these problems but decided to hold off from taking medications. I noticed over time, however, that the heart palpitations had increased. I had experienced these episodes on and off for two years, and in spite of efforts on my part (like discontinuing all caffeinated drinks and taking yoga) the anxiety episodes persisted. I was particularly concerned to notice that my resting heart rate—when I was doing non-strenuous activities like driving a car—was in the range of 100 to 120 beats per minute. The ringing in my ears had also become worse. At this point, I decided to try alternative healing at the East West Clinic before taking medications.

I received acupuncture therapy approximately once a week and took Chinese herbal pills for the ringing in the ears and the palpitations. I noticed an immediate decrease in my symptoms, especially during the first few treatments. However, the heart palpitations and generalized anxiety never completely left me. I would feel better for one to two days but then the anxiety and palpitations would return.

On April 19, 1994, at my regularly scheduled visit, the therapist reevaluated my progress and suggested that I take the questionnaire to rule out systemic Candida infection. I scored eight or more on the scale, which pointed to an affirmation that the reason I was not responding fully to therapy was that I had CRC. She had noticed that I had raised, white rashes in the skin of my neck, which looked to her like rashes indicative of Candida infestation. She explained that the presence of fungus in my system could be the reason why the energy balancing she was doing was not holding.

She told me to spend the next week understanding more about Candida Related Complex (CRC) and then decide whether I wanted to try the suggested regimen for treatment of the Candida. She gave me a book, *The Yeast*

Connection, to read. She also gave me handouts on the recommended diet and the information regarding the fungicide and colon cleansers I must take. These consisted of Caprol, bentonite, psyllium, and acidophilus. That week I read with interest all the material she gave me. I started following the diet and noted that I felt somewhat better. As a test, after I had followed the diet for a few days, I had a meal that included a glass of wine, steak with mushrooms, au gratin potatoes, and bread. That same night and on into the next day I felt ill and the heart palpitations intensified. This convinced me more than anything that there was a basis for this type of diet. I went back on the yeast-free, sugar-free recommended diet and again I felt the difference right away.

At my April 25th appointment I informed the acupuncturist that I was ready to start the colon cleansing program. Within the first week I noted significant improvement. I was very encouraged. The episodes of anxiety had decreased and for short periods of time I felt totally calm, a feeling I had not experienced in years. I did find the anxiety episodes more difficult to deal with once I experienced the calm and this motivated me to stay with the program. I did my yoga exercises more regularly as well as relaxation techniques, like meditation, self-healing tapes, and positive self-talk. I found as time went on that following the program became easier and I was gradually returning to my old self and was able to cope with stress.

During the first three weeks on the Acu-Trol program of colon cleansing, I noted some of the most dramatic changes. The frequency and intensity of the anxiety and palpitations had markedly decreased and my resting heart rate while driving a car came down to 70 to 90 beats per minute. The skin of my neck had gotten smoother. I had always thought that my rough skin texture was normal since I had the same skin texture since my teen years. There were also brown colored "age spots" that covered my arms, and, to my delight, these too had lightened up. My right ear had always felt like there was fluid build-up in it and this sensation had dissipated. Even the chronic achiness in my joints went away, along with the burning sensation I often felt in my feet. Overall, my moods were less erratic and the periods of depression had become less frequent. My energy was at an appropriate level without the dreaded periods of high anxiety. Also, the frequent hot flashes which disturbed my sleep went away.

After three weeks, my husband and daughter both commented that I glowed. I continue to take the Acu-Trol program and have continued to feel better, though the symptoms are diminishing at a slower rate than at first. I am also noticing that my problems with intestinal upsets are less frequent. I continue to take acupuncture sessions though less frequently, and the treatments are now holding.

It has been four months since I started treatments at the East West Clinic. In addition to the changes in my physical symptoms, I have also noticed a change in my mental outlook. Over the winter, I had made the decision to quit my job, which I had found to be very stressful, and had set my last working date as September 30, 1994. I now have more energy and find it easier to do the things my job requires. Also, since I am once again sleeping well, I am not arriving to work exhausted. I have a more positive attitude about my work and the 40 women I supervise. I no longer plan to leave my job in the near future, and I am enjoying the challenges and contacts that I am able to make in my work, rather than fearing them as I used to.

Moreover, I am pleased to note that I no longer have the incapacitating fear of speaking before a group. For as long as I can remember, even as far back as high school, I had a fear of speaking to groups. In spite of strategies that I used to keep my voice steady, it would always quiver, and I would lose my ability to think on the spot. Now, I am more assertive and am finding that my comments are more readily acknowledged. I feel that I am more respected.

When I first realized that these treatments were indeed on the right track for me, I talked to my 21-year-old daughter, who was having acute episodes of anxiety attacks. She was a few months away from graduation and I had planned to just wait until she had finished school before I encouraged her to get on the treatment program. However, since my recovery seemed to come so fast, I decided not to wait. So I suggested that she too start the evaluation and treatment for candidiasis right away.

I feel that the combination of the four treatments (Acu-Trol program, acupuncture, diet, and relaxation techniques) have been the right combination to control the chronic anxiety and depression I suffered for many years. It has also helped me cope better with my job and family responsibilities.

I have to pinpoint when the symptoms may have started for me and what I may have done to cause the Candida overgrowth. I recall having anxiety symptoms as a teenager and they got worse over the years. They became exacerbated when I got my current position, which is very stressful. I have not used antibiotics frequently; as a matter of fact, I did not use them at all from the time I was 21 years old until age 43. Neither have I used cortisone. I did grow up on a dairy farm, and my family drank a lot of milk. Possibly there were antibiotics in the milk we drank, as this was less regulated in the 1950s and 1960s. I also used birth control pills for a period of five to six months at age 21. I am not sure which triggered the overgrowth for me, but I now realize that I have had it for a long time and am very pleased to have found a clinic that was able to point me in the right direction to treat this very debilitating condition.

—Ann Bajari, Annandale, Minnesota

Chapter Four

Symptoms of Candida Related Complex

Symptoms which point toward Candida Related Complex (CRC) can be many and varied. CRC can be evaluated through a self-administered questionnaire. Some alternative health care providers feel that this type of questionnaire can be as accurate in analyzing symptoms as laboratory blood tests and/or stool cultures. If a high rating results, anti-fungal treatment is recommended.

A significant aspect of CRC is that it exacerbates any existing malady. Once a particular body system is disrupted and there is an overgrowth of fungi, the fungi easily invades the specific part of the victim's body which is weakest. For example, if a person has suffered from asthma, sinusitis, and allergies, they will probably experience these illnesses in a more intense and more frequent manner. Or if a person has been afflicted by occasional bladder infections, this urinary problem will magnify under the strain of CRC, and they will probably experience more frequent and severe bladder infections which can even escalate into kidney infections.

And unfortunately, if the illness is allowed to progress, additional symptoms will often appear in other body systems. In the example previously noted of the sufferer of frequent urinary infections, this person could continue to experience the initial bladder/kidney infections, but may also suffer from bronchial infections. Another example: if a person has suffered from repeated upper respiratory infections, while also battling pneumonia/bronchial infections, this person could begin to experience cardiovascular problems such as angina, arrhythmia, and strokes.

These CRC sufferers thus claim to perpetually be sick. No matter what they use to treat their symptoms, nothing seems to help. It is only after a careful analysis and study of each individual's illness history that the symptoms are pieced together to fit the elusive pattern characteristic of CRC.

Internist Leo Galland, M.D., summarized data on 91 patients with CRC. The percentages of patients reporting specific symptoms were as follows:

91%   reported fatigue
86%   reported food intolerance
81%   reported gastrointestinal disturbances
71%   reported alcohol intolerance
61%   reported chronic vaginitis
55%   reported poor memory
54%   reported depression
46%   reported chemical hypersensitivity
44%   reported PMS
39%   reported anxiety
29%   reported headaches
19%   reported carbohydrate cravings [1]

Note that fatigue is the most commonly reported symptom of CRC, with food intolerance and abdominal disturbances following close behind.

In 1980, CRC patient Lawrence A. Plumlee, M.D., wrote that intestinal gas, either in the form of flatulence or belching, occurs when undigested food stays in the intestines. [2] While remaining in the intestines, this undigested food feeds the intestinal flora, such as bacteria and fungi, which in turn produce alcohols and gas-containing hydrocarbons. This could explain why CRC patients experience improved health with the aid of anti-fungal medications that kill yeast and molds.

The presence of these by-products could also explain the rationale behind chemical sensitivities and food allergies. The undigested food, in conjunction with the alcohols and gas-producing hydrocarbons, travel into the bloodstream, causing allergies. Allergies develop from an improper immune system reaction to foreign bodies. Our immune system, designed to help fight infection, can wrongly identify a non-toxic substance. Then the white blood cells overreact and can actually inflict more damage than the invading foreign substance. [3] Dr. Plumlee also notes that if candida toxins enter the bloodstream, then the immune system overreacts to them, causing new food allergies to develop. These changes in the immune system produced by fungi result in problematic food and chemical sensitivities.

In addition to the allergies caused by CRC, these patients also experience physical problems because of a toxin that CRC produces. Orian Truss, M.D., one of the pioneers in the study of CRC, has a hypothesis regarding yeast and acetaldehyde. [4] Sugar is fermented causing ethanol. The fungi then metabolize ethanol to acetaldehyde. "Yeast are able to metabolize ethanol to acetaldehyde if oxygen is available . . . Indirect evidence indicates that, in vivo, Candida albicans ferments sugars to acetaldehyde." Symptoms of the presence of acetaldehyde are abdominal distention, excess flatus, and belching.

Causes of many major illnesses have puzzled physicians and medical researchers since they began studying diseases. Mycotoxin expert A.V. Constantini, M.D., is quoted in the World Health Organization (WHO) *Mycotoxins in Human Health Newsletter* as warning, "The data presented . . . points to our need to more fully appreciate the role of fungi and mycotoxins in the etiology (origin) of the major human diseases which have for so long remained a mystery as to their cause." [5] Now some scientists believe that fungi and the toxins they produce are the cause of major diseases.

In another study conducted by Dr. Constantini, fungi are implicated as the cause of many serious illnesses. These include a number of malignancies to organs including the esophagus, lung, colon, kidney, breast, uterus, blood, lymph nodes, brain and skin. [6] Some autoimmune diseases were also found to be caused by fungi. These include: Scleroderma (a thickening of skin especially on arms, hands and face, puffy hands and feet in morning, and joint pain and stiffness), diabetes (excessive urine excretion), rheumatoid arthritis (joint disorder), Sjogren's syndrome (red, gritty eyes), psoriasis (red, scaly skin), and systemic lupus erythematosus (skin lesions). Fungi and the toxins they produce have also been documented as the cause of gout (sudden, severe joint pain with swelling and redness) and hyperuricemia (excessive uric acid in the blood). The following cardiovascular diseases have also been documented to be caused by fungi and their toxins: atherosclerosis (cholesterol deposits in the arteries), hyperlipidemia (excess of fats in the blood), angina, myocardial infarction (heart muscle dies due to blockage of blood supply), arrhythmia (irregular heartbeat), carotid artery occlusion (neck artery blockage), stroke, intermittent claudication (cramping of leg muscles), and gangrene.

Dr. Constantini also listed other assumed fungal-mycotoxin-caused glandular and muscle-related diseases: Raynaud's Syndrome (contraction of arteries causing fingers and toes to turn white upon exposure to cold or emotion), shoulder-hand syndrome, sarcoidosis (benign tumors in any part of the body but especially in the lungs), Duchenne's muscular dystrophy (muscle weakness, progressive crippling), precocious (unusually early) puberty in boys, and Cushing's Disease (excess secretion of adrenal hormone). Dr. Constantini has shown that fungi and their resulting toxins can cause cancer and autoimmune diseases, and adversely affect our cardiovascular system, glands, and hormones. Thus, fungus, by weakening our immune system, can cause a multiplicity of serious illnesses.

A study of a self-administered questionnaire as an aid to diagnosing CRC was published in *The Journal of Advancement in Medicine*. [7] This study compared four self-administered questionnaires to laboratory blood tests, vaginal cultures, and antibody assay (analysis) levels in diagnosing CRC. Four self-tests were used in this study: Dr. Crook's Yeast Questionnaire; Cornell Index; Beck Index; and Type A Score. Three of the four self-administered questionnaires, the first three respectively, proved to be equally accurate as blood tests, cultures, and assays. The results showed that:

> There was good correlation between the results of three questionnaires (Candida Questionnaire included) and the laboratory tests. If the results of this test (lab tests) were high, so were (three of the four) self-test scores . . . The results obtained were also of use in monitoring the clinical progress of the patients. As their clinical status improved, both the questionnaire scores and lab results showed substantial declines.

The questionnaire proved accurate in diagnosing CRC when the results were compared to lab tests, cultures, and assays. It is clear that Dr. Crook's self-administered Candida questionnaire can be of significant value in the diagnostic screening and follow-up progress for CRC.

The following is a questionnaire by John Trowbridge, M.D. [8]

"Rate Your Health" Quiz for the Yeast Syndrome

There are several ways you can privately determine at home whether you have been affected by Candida albicans. The most important question that you might ask yourself or that you may be asked by your doctor is: "When was the last time that I (you) felt well?" Added to that very basic piece of information should be responses to Dr. Trowbridge's "Rate Your Health Quiz." Take the quiz and learn if you may need treatment for Candida illness.

Circle the number of the question to which you must answer "yes." If you have four or five "yes" answers, you may suffer with yeast-related illness; if you have six or seven "yes" answers, you probably are a Candida infection victim; if you have eight or more "yes" answers, you almost certainly need medical treatment for chronic generalized candidiasis or for unusual illnesses that occasionally mimic the condition and for which proper medical diagnosis and care should be sought.

Questions for Adults and Teenagers

Have you suffered from:
1. Frequent infections, constant skin problems—or taken antibiotics (or cortisone medications) often or for long periods?
2. Feelings of fatigue, being drained of energy, or drowsiness—or the same symptoms on damp muggy days, or in moldy places such as basements?
3. Feelings of anxiety, irritability, insomnia—cravings for sugary foods, breads, or alcoholic beverages?
4. Food sensitivities, allergy reactions—or digestion problems, bloating, heartburn, constipation, or bad breath?
5. Feeling "spacy" or "unreal," difficulty in concentration, or being bothered by perfumes, chemical fumes, or tobacco smoke?
6. Poor coordination, muscle weakness, or painful or swollen joints?
7. Mood swings, depression, or loss of sexual feelings?
8. Dry mouth or throat, nose congestion or drainage, pressure above or behind the eyes or ears, or frequent headaches?
9. Pains in the chest, shortness of breath, dizziness or easy bruising?
10. Frustration of going from doctor to doctor, never getting your health completely well—or being told that your symptoms are "mental" or "psychological" or "psychosomatic"?

For Women Only

Have you suffered from:
1. Vaginal burning or itching, discharge, or infections—or urinary problems?
2. A difficult time getting pregnant—or been pregnant two or more times, or taken birth control pills?

3. Premenstrual symptoms: moodiness, fluid loading, tension, irregular cycles or other menstrual or sexual problems?

Especially for Children

Have you suffered from:
1. Frequent infections, particularly of the ears, tonsilitis, bronchitis, or history of frequent diaper rash?
2. Continuous nasal congestion or drainage?
3. Dark circles under the eyes, periods of hyperactivity, or poor attention span?

By reviewing the Candida Questionnaire, one sees how numerous and varied the symptoms of CRC can be. This information-gathering tool evaluates specific physical symptoms to determine the presence and extent of CRC. People afflicted with this disease will not necessarily have all the symptoms listed; CRC may focus its damage on just one organ or system. If the patient checks a significant number of symptoms, then an analysis of the questionnaire should be made, along with an examination of the patient's history. If the questionnaire responses are in the high range or even if symptoms are few but have been persistent (occurring for six months or more), then the conclusion can be supported that there is a need for treatment.

The following is Dr. Crook's self-administered questionnaire: [9]

Dr. Crook's Yeast Questionnaire and Score Sheet

Dr. Trowbridge has also utilized the Candida Questionnaire and Score Sheet (the Y-score) as developed and described by William G. Crook, M.D., of Jackson, Tennessee, in his book *The Yeast Connection*. This questionnaire is often provided as a diagnostic tool by Candida-conscious physicians as part of recording the patient's health history. An inquiring doctor then is able quickly to evaluate the likely role of Candida albicans in contributing to illness.

Dr. Crook's yeast questionnaire gives additional scoring emphasis to a patient's answers in the following categories that are the source of, or are often associated with, yeast-related illness:

1. Taking antibiotics such as tetracyclines, sulfas and sulfa combinations, synthetic penicillins, and other "broad spectrum" antibiotics.
2. Taking birth control pills or having been pregnant.
3. Taking cortisone or other steroid medications.
4. Having "chemical sensitivities" or other significant allergy problems.
5. Reacting to molds, fungi, yeast, and other parasites.
6. Craving sweets, alcohol, or breads.
7. Frequently feeling the wide variety of symptoms noted at the beginning of this chapter.

The patient's scores are totaled to determine whether there is a symptomatic relationship to yeast disease. A yeast questionnaire also exists for children, which Dr. Crook has made a part of another small book that he published in 1984.

Review of Personal Health Problems and Concerns

A full review of your own clinical history is a critical part in the correct approach to ascertaining whether you are the unwilling host for expanding colonics of yeast organisms. Your present feelings and observations about yourself are every bit as valuable as any laboratory or physical examination. Your physician will want to know what you sense about your body's functions and how your mind and emotions are working. *The Review of Personal Health Problems and Concerns* supplied below can be an important tool for you and your health professional. It was adapted by Dr. Trowbridge from an earlier symptom survey form distributed by Standard Process Laboratories, Milwaukee, Wisconsin.

Although extensively used by doctors for diagnostic purposes, this evaluation form is not necessarily a physician's patient history document. Rather, it's a patient self-testing technique. You are creating a diagnostic tool in your own home when you have the time and opportunity to reflect on your discomforts. Seeing, for instance, that you have thyroid stress or adrenal stress, a health professional trained in holistic approaches to healing illness will be more efficiently able to counsel you. This will save you time, discomfort, and money. You will need less testing from the beginning because fewer areas will have to be examined.

Do the following:

1. Use a pen and mark in the space provided your numbered point score to the question asked, if the question fits what you have been experiencing.
2. Mark only the signs, symptoms, or complaints that apply specifically to you; leave all others unmarked.
3. Use the number codes of 1, 2, or 3 for scoring your answers, placing your assessment score on the line between the question and the question's number.

Write "3" for problems you notice every day or at least once a week.
Write "2" for problems you notice about once or twice a month.
Write "1" for problems you notice irregularly or occasionally.

I. Sympathetic Nervous System Function

1. _____ "Lump" in throat
2. _____ Dry mouth, eyes, or nose
3. _____ Strong light irritates eyes
4. _____ Gag easily
5. _____ Body temperature easily raised
6. _____ Arms or legs cold or clammy
7. _____ "Goose bumps" common
8. _____ Staring, blink little
9. _____ Pulse speeds up after meals
10. _____ Heart pounds after retiring

11. _____ "Keyed up"—can't relax
12. _____ Jumpy, mind overly active
13. _____ Burning, tingling, or sharp pains
14. _____ Cuts heal slowly
15. _____ Urine amount reduced
16. _____ Cold sweats often
17. _____ Appetite reduced
18. _____ Acid foods upset stomach
19. _____ "Nervous" stomach
20. _____ Sour stomach often

Related problems not mentioned above: _____
_____
_____

II. Parasympathetic Nervous System Function

1. _____ Joint stiffness after arising
2. _____ Muscle cramps in legs and toes at night
3. _____ Perspire easily
4. _____ Watery eyes or nose
5. _____ Eyes blink often
6. _____ Eyelids swollen or puffy
7. _____ Hoarseness
8. _____ Breathing irregular
9. _____ Slow or irregular pulse
10. _____ Difficulty swallowing
11. _____ Need to eat often or feel hunger pains, faintness
12. _____ Indigestion soon after meals
13. _____ Stomach growling or churning
14. _____ Vomit easily or frequently
15. _____ "Butterfly" stomach or cramps
16. _____ Alternating constipation and diarrhea
17. _____ Circulation poor or hands or feet sensitive to cold
18. _____ Slow reflexes
19. _____ Easily get colds, bronchitis, or asthma

Related problems not mentioned above: _____
_____
_____

III. Adrenal System Function

1. _____ Pounding headaches
2. _____ Tendency to higher blood pressure
3. _____ "Hot flashes"
4. _____ Dizziness sensations
5. _____ Exhaustion or can't cope
6. _____ Constant fatigue
7. _____ Tend to have lower blood pressure
8. _____ Circulation poor in hands or feet
9. _____ Abnormal sweating
10. _____ History of kidney trouble or swelling ankles
11. _____ Crave salt or salty foods
12. _____ Brown spots or bronzing of skin
13. _____ Nails weak or have ridges
14. _____ (Women) Masculine body traits
15. _____ (Women) Hair growth on face or body
16. _____ History of sugar in urine but not diagnosed with diabetes
17. _____ Weakness or dizziness
18. _____ Joint or arthritis-like pain
19. _____ Tend to have hives or welts
20. _____ Tend to have allergies or asthma
21. _____ Frequent or continuing colds or infections
22. _____ Weakness prolonged after colds or flu

Related problems not mentioned above: _____

_____

_____

IV. Cardiovascular/Respiratory System Functions

1. _____ Aware of "breathing heavily"
2. _____ Want to open windows when in closed rooms
3. _____ Sigh often—"hunger for air"
4. _____ High altitude causes discomfort
5. _____ Shortness of breath with increased activity
6. _____ Dull pressure or pain in chest or left arm, worse with increased activity
7. _____ "Tightness" in chest that becomes worse with increased activity

8. _____ Muscle cramps that become worse with exercise—"charley horses"

9. _____ Hands or feet "go to sleep" or feel tingling or numbness

10. _____ Swollen ankles that are worse in the evening

11. _____ Bruise easily

12. _____ Nose bleeds easily

13. _____ History of anemia or low blood count

14. _____ Noises or "ringing" in ears

15. _____ Easily get colds or fevers

16. _____ Afternoon "yawner"

17. _____ Get drowsy during day or early evening

Related problems not mentioned above: _____

_____

_____

V. Thyroid Gland Function

1. _____ Insomnia or too easily awakened

2. _____ Nervousness or anxiety

3. _____ Highly emotional

4. _____ Inward trembling

5. _____ Irritable and restless

6. _____ Heart pounds or skips

7. _____ Pulse fast at rest

8. _____ Increase in weight

9. _____ Decreased appetite

10. _____ Sleepy during day

11. _____ Mental sluggishness

12. _____ Fatigue easily

13. _____ Headaches upon arising that wear off during day

14. _____ "Get up and go" has "got up and gone"

15. _____ Night sweats

16. _____ Flush easily

17. _____ Feel drained in heat

18. _____ Thin (unpadded) or moist skin

19. _____ Eyelids and face twitch

20. _____ Can't work under pressure

21. _____ Increased appetite
22. _____ Can't gain weight
23. _____ Slow pulse
24. _____ Poor hearing
25. _____ Noises or "ringing" in ears
26. _____ Frequent urination
27. _____ Hair coarse or falls out easily
28. _____ Dry or scaly skin
29. _____ Constipation or hard stools
30. _____ Sensitive to cold

Related problems not mentioned above: _____

_____

_____

VI. Sugar-Handling Ability

1. _____ Hungry between meals
2. _____ Irritable or moody before meals
3. _____ Get "shaky" when hungry
4. _____ Faintness when meals delayed
5. _____ Fatigue relieved by food
6. _____ Heart pounds or skips when meals missed or delayed
7. _____ Afternoon or late morning headaches
8. _____ Awaken after few hours of sleep—hard to return to sleep
9. _____ Abnormal craving for sweets or snacks between meals and at bedtime
10. _____ Crave candy, coffee, tea, or cola in afternoon
11. _____ Overeating sweets upsets body or mind
12. _____ Appetite excessive
13. _____ Eat when nervous or upset
14. _____ Moods of depression or melancholy

Related problems not mentioned above: _____

_____

_____

VII. Pituitary Gland Function

1. _____ Failing memory
2. _____ "Splitting" headaches in forehead or temples

3. _____ Excessive thirst

4. _____ Weight gain around hips or waist

5. _____ Feel better after eating sweets

6. _____ Have lower blood pressure

7. _____ Increased sexual desire

8. _____ Sexual desire reduced or lacking

9. _____ Sugar-handling problems

10. _____ Tend to have ulcers or bowel problems

11. _____ Bloating of intestines

Related problems not mentioned above: _____

_____

_____

VIII. A. Liver and Gall Bladder Function

1. _____ Bitter, metallic taste in mouth in the morning

2. _____ Stools that float or form an "oil slick" on water in toilet

3. _____ Stools light brown, tan, or gray

4. _____ Greasy foods cause digestive upset

5. _____ Pains in upper right belly after eating

6. _____ Pains behind right shoulder or right shoulder blade

7. _____ Bowel movements painful or difficult

8. _____ Laxatives needed for regularity

9. _____ Stools alternate between firm and watery

10. _____ Blurred vision

11. _____ Burning feet

12. _____ Skin peels on soles of feet

13. _____ History of gall bladder attacks or gall stones

14. _____ Dry skin

15. _____ Skin rashes

16. _____ Itchy skin or feet

17. _____ Hair falling out excessively

VIII. B. Allergy Interrelated with Liver System Function

18. _____ Dizziness

19. _____ Nightmares

20. _____ Sneezing attacks

21. _____ Bad breath or "halitosis"
22. _____ Milk, milk products, or cheese cause distress
23. _____ Crave sweets
24. _____ Feel drained in hot weather
25. _____ Burning or itching anus
26. _____ Hemorrhoid problems

Related problems not mentioned above: _____

_____

_____

IX. Gastrointestinal Function From Stomach to Anus

1. _____ Burning stomach relieved by eating
2. _____ Dark tar-like color to stools
3. _____ Indigestion one-half to one hour after eating (or may occur in three or four hours)
4. _____ Gas or rumbling shortly after eating
5. _____ Stomach "bloating" after eating
6. _____ Loss of taste for meat
7. _____ Coated tongue
8. _____ Lower bowel gas several hours after eating
9. _____ Stools have foul odor
10. _____ Stools lumpy or hard—constipation
11. _____ Stools runny or watery—diarrhea
12. _____ Mucus mixed with stools
13. _____ Blood mixed with stools

Related problems not mentioned above: _____

_____

_____

X. A. For Women Only

1. _____ Premenstrual tension
2. _____ Premenstrual swelling or "puffiness"
3. _____ Depressed feelings before menses
4. _____ Very easily fatigued
5. _____ Painful menses
6. _____ Menses excessive and prolonged

7. _____ Menses usually closer than twenty-six days

8. _____ Painful breasts

9. _____ Sexual desire reduced or lacking

10. _____ Vaginal discharge

11. _____ Had hysterectomy with both ovaries removed

12. _____ Menopause—"hot flashes" or mood changes

13. _____ Menses scanty or missed

14. _____ Acne worse at menses

15. _____ Melancholy, sadness, or depression

16. _____ History of kidney or urine infections or blood in urine

Related problems not mentioned above: _____

_____

_____

X. B. For Men Only

1. _____ Feeling of incomplete emptying of bowels

2. _____ Urination two or more times per night

3. _____ Urination difficult or with dribbling

4. _____ History of prostate trouble

5. _____ Pain on inside of legs or heels

6. _____ Legs jerking or restless in bed at night

7. _____ History of kidney or urine infections or blood in urine

8. _____ Tire too easily

9. _____ Lack of energy

10. _____ Avoid physical activity

11. _____ Melancholy, sadness, or depression

12. _____ Aches and pains that seem to move around the body

13. _____ Sexual desire reduced or gone

Related problems not mentioned above: _____

_____

_____

Score yourself for the yeast syndrome. Here is what your numbered scorings mean:

Any group in which you score fifteen points or more, you must consider that candidiasis might be causing problems in that body system.

Any group in which you score ten to fourteen points, you should consider that candidiasis possibly contributes to problems in that body system.

Any group in which you score less than ten points but you've marked several answers with the number 3 or 2, consider that candidiasis may be weakening that body system.

In fact, pay attention to any individual 3 response. This higher number will alert your physician to check more closely that particular body tissue, part, organ, or system for effects of yeast infestation or other disturbance to healthy function.

A total score for the entire questionnaire is not relevant. *The Review of Personal Health Problems and Concerns* does not work that way. You may be exceedingly affected in one area and not at all in another. These are actually ten small health history tests, which together indicate a pattern of illness for evaluation by your holistic physician. Traditionally practicing physicians could also find your information valuable, directing them to look more closely at areas of health problems for you that previously had been ignored or simply skipped over in earlier evaluations.

With the aid of these self-administered questionnaires, the challenge for the skilled practitioner, or the informed patient for that matter, is to piece the symptoms together to discover if these symptoms point to CRC. The clues are first picked up during the initial intake interview process, where the practitioner and/or informed patient carefully assesses the symptoms, reviews the patient's history, observes the current manifestations, and arrives at the initial assessment of CRC. Based on the assessment and confirmed by a high scoring in the self-administered questionnaire, the treatment is started at once.

In conclusion, the symptoms of CRC are legion and varied. Screening for CRC can be done by physical exam, laboratory tests and/or a self-administered questionnaire.

Chapter Five

The Professional Controversy

In the late 1970s, Candida Related Complex (CRC) was discovered and quickly gained recognition as an illness that affects a great many people. Even though the general public accepted and recognized CRC, the medical establishment did not. This was in spite of evidence that CRC was an illness that could have serious consequences if not addressed.

In 1977, information written by Orian Truss, M.D., was published in the *Journal of Orthomolecular Medicine*. [1] Then in 1983, his associate William Crook, M.D., mentioned this problem on a television program in Cincinnati, Ohio. Dr. Crook was deluged with over 7,300 letters the following week from CRC sufferers. Realizing that there were many more people affected than had previously been recognized, Dr. Crook wrote a book entitled *The Yeast Connection*, which has since sold more than 1.4 million copies.

In spite of the fact that the book has been so well received by the general public, the American Academy of Allergy and Immunology (AAAI), the American Medical Association (AMA), and the Food and Drug Administration (FDA) are unwilling to recognize this illness. Dr. Truss feels that, "The very complexity of its (CRC's) manifestations is perhaps the greatest single obstacle to acceptance of the concept that Candida albicans may be responsible for chronic illness." [2] It is, in fact, the myriad symptoms of CRC which offer this illness its very cloak.

Ignoring the public's interest in and acceptance of CRC, the AAAI issued a statement in the *Journal of Allergy and Clinical Immunology* in 1986 (nine years after the release of *The Yeast Connection*) stating:

> On the basis of the evidence so far reviewed and until appropriate published evidence to the contrary is brought to its attention, the Practice Standards Committee recommends that the concept of the candidiasis hypersensitivity syndrome is unproven. [3]

This position statement was signed and approved by the eleven all-male (Eighty percent of CRC patients are women and children) AAAI executive committee. Many alternative health care providers and knowledgeable lay people have a problem with the phrase "until appropriate published evidence to the contrary is brought to its attention." In fact, since 1986, many studies published (some as early as 1964), in both American and European medical journals, have been brought to their attention. To date, the AAAI still has not revised this position paper.

In addition to the AAAI decision, a second obstacle to CRC's gaining medical acceptance was presented — this time by the AMA. In September of 1987, in the *Journal of the American Medical Association*, the AMA issued a very similar statement, again using the phrase "candidiasis hypersensitivity syndrome is unproven." [4] Subsequently, a third impediment occurred when the Food and Drug Administration (FDA) adopted the same stance with the identical wording in their October, 1989 *FDA Consumer* magazine. [5]

This "unproven" stance on CRC by some medical and governmental organizations continues even though results of more than 100 studies proving CRC have been presented to them.

Since these position papers have been published, CRC patients are often unable to receive insurance coverage for their medical expenses. Furthermore, the FDA is trying to take many harmless and quite beneficial products off the market. These products are dietary supplements and anti-fungal products, which are needed by CRC patients.

Readers of *Family Circle* magazine, in an article entitled "Hazardous Health Cures," were asked to report the names of doctors who treat CRC to the National Council Against Health Fraud (NCAHF). The authors stated that CRC was a "hot allergy-related scam." The information in the magazine nearly replicated the information in the FDA publication. [6] As a result, one member of the NCAHF committee testified under oath that they have a list of 40,000 health providers on his computer whom he suspects of using questionable medical practices. [7]

These position statements regarding CRC by the AAAI, AMA, and FDA have been used by the NCAHF to intimidate doctors who might otherwise be willing to help CRC patients. The repercussions of these nearly identical statements cause doctors treating CRC to fear the loss of their medical licenses by a peer-review committee. Physicians have been called before their state medical licensing boards and forced to hire expensive legal representation. Some have lost the license to practice or have had tens of thousands of dollars of insurance reimbursement withheld. These physicians are harassed by their state boards for treating patients with illnesses considered "unproven."

The National Institutes of Health (NIH), on the other hand, realizes that CRC needs to be researched. In 1990, NIH granted the University of Cincinnati (UC) Medical Center a $3.75 million five-year grant to study fungal infections. Under the direction of Dr. Ward Bullock, director of UC's infectious disease division, this grant is designed to study the fundamentals of fungal infections. "As we become more sophisticated at suppressing the immune system," Dr. Bullock says, "we greatly increase the risk of serious infection." This study delves into how the fungi spread, how to better diagnose fungal infections, and how to find more effective and less toxic drugs to treat these infections. An understanding of how a healthy immune system fights the infections is also essential. The UC researchers are focusing on four fungi that are fairly recognizable to the general public:

1. Aspergillus, a common bread mold. In humans, this fungus can appear first in the lungs, imitating pneumonia;
2. Candida, little understood beyond vaginal yeast infections in women;
3. Histoplasma, a lung infection that can result in a chest-cold-like illness in healthy people but that will not go away in people with suppressed immune systems. This fungus infects about half a million Midwesterners annually, though not all get seriously ill.
4. Pneumocystic carinii, which causes the pneumonia-like illness that kills most AIDS patients.

"We know so little about them (these fungi) that research is critical," Dr. Bullock says. "We've got to raise medical awareness of these organisms."

Previously both Washington University in St. Louis and the University of California at Los Angeles have received prestigious fungus grants from NIH. Clearly, NIH realizes fungus is a problem affecting humans that deserves further study. [8]

Although awareness of CRC is beginning to be evidenced by some U.S. health care professionals, we are decades behind other countries. In 1974, a Russian mycologist (one who studies fungi), P.N. Kasckin, M.D., published a major review of the literature in the *Journal of Mycopathologia et Mycologia*. Heavily referenced with 94 citations, this article summarized research on CRC for the 10 years between 1964 and 1974.

Dr. Kasckin listed eleven forms of allergic lesions, sensitization to antibiotic drugs, and also mentions the chronic form of candidiasis. In his paper, he also cites many factors not usually associated with causing CRC, including x-ray therapy, air pollution, and detergents. Dr. Kasckin also cites many symptoms resulting from CRC, such as the breakage of vitamin metabolism, asthma, thrombophlebitis, and psoriasis, to name a few. His paper also mentions that mixed infections (fungal, viral, and bacterial) are the most difficult type to diagnose. [9]

What is surprising to U.S. readers is that this data was published years ago, some as early as 1964! Obviously, since other researchers recognized CRC long before their U.S. counterparts, the European pool of information is much greater than in America. Hopefully, the AAAI, AMA, and FDA will examine the published literature and issue an amended position statement on CRC.

Now new light has been shed in the U.S. by a 1993 study which was reported in the *New England Journal of Medicine*. The report surprised mainstream medicine, but not the average American. The study proved that an unexpectedly high number of our citizens were seeing alternative therapists for help with their health problems (including CRC), and that they were receiving assistance that their regular doctors were not providing. The article reported on the use and frequency of unconventional medicine. Unconventional medicine refers to medical practices that are "not in conformity with the standards of the medical community." Many other people simply refer to this therapy as alternative medicine. Alternative medicine works with the body's healing systems, enhancing natural defenses rather than suppressing symptoms. Complementary medicine would be a more appropriate term in light of the fact that more than half of those visiting alternative therapists also saw a medical doctor. In fact, these two forms of treatment — conventional and alternative — can complement each other.

Researchers involved in this study wanted to know overall prevalence, cost and patterns of use of this type of therapy. Prior to the study, the researchers assumed an estimated prevalence of use of unconventional therapy at between 10% and 50% of the population. Information was gleaned from telephone interviews with 1,539 adults. One in three respondents (or 34%) replied that they used at least one unconventional therapy in the past year. Researchers discovered that the estimated total number of annual visits made to alternative therapists in 1990 topped 425 million. This figure was one-third of the respondents and reflects 12% of the adult population. This number is greater than the number of annual visits to medical doctors, including all primary care medical doctors nationwide.

The frequency of use of unconventional therapy is much higher than medical personnel had suspected. The reason for lack of awareness is that most of those who visit alternative therapists do not inform their medical doctors. However, 89% said that they visited an alternative therapist without the recommendation of a doctor.

"Who were the people who sought alternative therapists?" the researchers asked. The study revealed that those who had a relatively higher level of education and a higher income were the individuals patronizing unconventional therapy: 44% had some college education; 39% had annual income above $35,000, and the age group consisted mainly of 25 to 49 year olds.

The cost of this alternative therapy amounted to $13.7 billion in 1990. Three-quarters of this amount was paid by the individual: 55% paid the entire cost themselves; a third-party (insurance) paid the remainder. Of the $13.7 billion spent for unconventional therapy, $11.7 billion went for the services of alternative therapists (assuming patients paid their bills in full). The other $2 billion was spent for nutritional supplements, books, and other materials. "The amount spent out-of-pocket on unconventional therapy was comparable to the amount spent out-of-pocket by Americans for all hospitalizations," the study reported.

The study revealed that the average American citizen believes that alternative medicine is useful for treating certain maladies, preventing illness, and maintaining optimal health.

The researchers reported, "We found that unconventional medicine has an enormous presence in the U.S. health care system." Additionally, they noted that "the (study) design may have resulted in an underestimate of the use of unconventional therapy" which means that probably an even greater number of people use alternative therapists than the study showed.

Since one person in three uses alternative therapy, according to the study, it is likely that all medical doctors, without realizing it, see patients who routinely use alternative therapies. The report suggested that, "perhaps medical doctors do not discuss the use of unconventional therapies because they lack adequate knowledge of these techniques."

This 1993 article suggested that the "newly established Office for the Study of Unconventional Medical Practices at the National Institute of Health (NIH) should help promote scholarly research and education in this area." [10]

There is more good news from the government for those interested in alternative medicine. On June 14, 1993, President William Clinton signed a law which established within the NIH an office to be known as the Office of Alternative Medicine (OAM). Its purpose is "to facilitate the evaluation of alternative medical treatment modalities, including acupuncture and Oriental medicine, homeopathic medicine, and physical manipulation therapies." Its duties are "to set up an information clearinghouse to exchange information with the public about alternative medicine (and) to support research training . . ." [11] Joseph Jacobs, M.D., original director of OAM, intends to create about 20 grants of $30,000. The grant categories are as follows: 1. diet, nutrition, and lifestyle; 2. mind/body control; 3. traditional and ethnomedicine; 4. structural manipulation and energetic therapies; 5. bioelectric applications; and 6. pharmacological and biological treatments.

Despite the fact that the general public and alternative health care providers recognize CRC, the AAAI, AMA, and FDA still have not. Hopefully, the published literature and the NIH will help these organizations accept the fact that CRC is an illness and many people are suffering and need help.

Case Study Three

47-Year-Old Male: Bronchial Infection

I am a 47-year-old husband and father of three and have been a Registered Nurse for 17 years. My primary symptoms were chest pain and hemoptysis (blood in the sputum).

In mid-August of 1993, while on a canoe/camping trip with my family, I was suddenly awakened with sharp, stabbing pains in the back of my lower left chest. Being a trained critical and emergency care nurse, I was able to determine that these pains were not signs of a heart attack but rather were coming from the lungs or the chest cavity.

The following day the pain had lessened in intensity, though I still had constant dull pain in the same area of my chest. Over the next several days, I became noticeably ill with weakness, fatigue, sweating, and coughing. At this point I decided to see my doctor. By the time I got to his office, I was coughing up green phlegm. He gave me antibiotics and sent me home. Within a week, the phlegm had turned rusty in color and there was frank bleeding (fresh blood).

Throughout the next three months, my health went through a harrowing roller-coaster of ups and downs. I would go to work for two weeks and then stay home for five days; this cycle went on and on. My strength was gradually diminishing and by mid-November I had become so fatigued that I had to cut back my work schedule. I was able to work only half a day at a time, and even then I had to spend many days recuperating from that half day of work. Fortunately, my employer was very supportive and allowed me to do only what I was able to do. Finally, in December I had to go on a short-term disability plan.

Meanwhile my medical doctors were stumped. Throughout my illness I had received standard and appropriate testing and treatment including sputum cultures, bronchoscopy, CAT scan, innumerable blood tests, and multiple antibiotic treatments. Early on, my primary physician referred me to a pulmonary specialist. Finally a team of doctors decided that I should undergo surgery for lung biopsy. The conclusion from all the testing, including the biopsy, was that there was nothing wrong with my lungs. The doctors were not certain as to the cause and how to proceed further with my treatment. Several rounds of antibiotic therapy did not work. I was still coughing up blood daily and still felt so fatigued that I was not able to contribute quality time as an employee or be effective as a father and as a husband.

Many times during my ordeal, friends had suggested that I try "alternative" forms of treatment, but I felt committed to stay with my own doctors. By late January 1994, five months after my initial bout with chest pain (with only a tentative diagnosis of bacterial infection and possible interstitial fibrosis with the recommendation to try massive doses of antibiotics), I felt it was time to give up and try something else. My short-term disability leave was coming to an end. Also, my marriage was strained to the point that it was seriously threatened.

Following the recommendation of a trusted friend, I went to see S. Colet Lahoz, RN, MS, an acupuncture therapist. At this time I was still having severe pleuritic pain in the left lower lobe as well as pain in the chest wall both back and front. The pain was often so bad it felt like I was hit with a baseball bat. She took a detailed history of my illness and then asked to see my tongue. Then she took my pulses. She said my lung channel showed a fast pulse with a wiry quality. She assessed this as indicative of "lung heat." She explained that "heat" in the lung channel caused irritation, phlegm formation, and inflammation. To balance this, she had to use acupuncture needles and herbal pills to "cool" the lung channel. In addition, she fine-tuned all the other channels in order to bring back harmony to my disrupted system.

She recommended that I see her twice a week at first and that we would taper the frequency of visits as I improved. On my second visit, she recommended that I take a multivitamin supplement with extra potassium and iron (KM by Matol) to help me regain my strength. She also asked that I take the test-yourself-questionnaire to rule out Candida related complex. She suspected this overgrowth as a possible outcome caused by the multiple use of antibiotics in recent months. Her hunch was right. I scored seven on the questionnaire, with three rated "persistent." This was enough to convince me that I should try cleaning out my system by using herbal fungicides and colon cleansers (products by Acu-Trol). She also suggested that I go on a yeast-free, sugar-free diet until the symptoms subsided.

The change was astounding! Within a week, I was able to return to my former work schedule. Over the next four weeks, I was able to gradually increase my work load. I progressed rapidly. Even when I did experience setbacks, they responded quickly to increased frequency of acupuncture treatments and herbal medicine. By the second month, the episodes of increased phlegm and hemoptysis were fewer and farther between. I also found out that the hemoptysis was very well controlled with acupuncture, Pinellia (a Chinese herbal formula for lung heat), and a combination of Echinacea and goldenseal herbs. The last two herbs act as natural antibiotics.

As my vigor returned to previous levels, I also noticed my sense of humor coming back. I did not realize how much I had missed laughter. I was able to concentrate better, think in the abstract, and think intelligently. The joy of walking and rough-housing with my boys is something I had forgotten and was glad to see return. Most of all, my wife Mary Jo and I were able to regain the warm and loving relationship we had lost. Recovery has saved my marriage!

With Colet's support and advice, I was brave enough to make major changes in my career in order to reduce stress and fatigue. Today, three and a half months since I started therapy with Colet at the East West Clinic, my life has finally returned to normal. I no longer need acupuncture treatments and, on Colet's advice, I continue to observe the recommended diet and take acidophilus. I also am back to exercising regularly. I anticipate full recovery by this summer.

I hope that my experience is not seen as a condemnation of Western physicians. I feel that their approach was appropriate and that I was always treated with respect. Rather, I hope that my story illustrates that so called "alternative therapies" have a valuable contribution to health care. In my case, it was the lifesaving solution to my problem.

I wish to express my sincere gratitude to Colet Lahoz for bringing me back from this condition and doing this with the perfect mixture of warmth, truthfulness, guidance, and friendship.

—Scott Bennett, RN, Stillwater, Minnesota

At this writing, January 1996 Scott Bennett continues to remain in good health and is working full time as a nurse. He had two or three minor exacerbations of coughing with greenish colored phlegm which was controlled by taking Echinasea and Goldenseal herbs.

Chapter Six

Mixed Infections as Part of the CRC Problem

Mixed gastrointestinal infections are part of the CRC problem. A weakened system is not able to resist parasitic fungi, bacteria, and worms. A parasite is any organism which feeds or lives on or in a different organism. Overexposure to antibiotics, through prescription drugs, ingesting meat from animals medicated with these drugs, contaminated water, travel which brings us in contact with parasites, household pets, parasites spread via daycare centers and unhealthy sexual practices all contribute to the increasing incidence of parasitic inhabitation of humans.

Mixed gastrointestinal infections are widespread even in technologically advanced countries. These infections begin mildly and at first can often be misdiagnosed as indigestion or exhaustion. If untreated, the situation intensifies and severe diarrhea begins with resultant malabsorption of nutrients and electrolyte disturbances.

These mixed infections have several names, including fungal/bacteria co-infection and intestinal dysbiosis. "Dysbiosis is a state of living with intestinal flora that has harmful effects," say internist Leo Galland, M.D., a specialist in nutrition and immunology, and naturopathic physician Stephen Barrie. They feel many more yeast and/or bacterial disease-producing microorganisms may be involved other than just Candida albicans. [1] This intestinal imbalance is due to either putrefactions, fermentations, deficiency of beneficial flora, and/or sensitization causing allergic reactions.

Putrefaction dysbiosis results from diets high in fat and animal flesh and low in soluble fiber. This condition results from the interplay of bacteria and diet and their effects on health and disease.

Fermentation is carbohydrate intolerance caused by an overgrowth of bacteria developing internally in the stomach, small intestine, and cecum. This gastric bacterial overgrowth increases the risk of systemic infection. British scientists have tentatively concluded that the majority of gut-fermentation cases are actually due to yeast overgrowth with only 20% attributed to bacterial imbalance. [2] Those afflicted with a fermentation problem experience abdominal distension, carbohydrate intolerance, fatigue, and impaired ability to think.

Deficiency of normal intestinal flora (good bacteria) can be caused by exposure to antibiotics, Galland believes, or a diet depleted of soluble fiber. This can result in food intolerance and a condition called irritable bowel syndrome (IBS). IBS patients suffer from excess secretion of mucus in stools, nausea, flatulence, bloating, anorexia, abdominal pain, constipation, and/or diarrhea.

Sensitization is an aggravation of normal immune response resulting in inflammatory bowel disease (infected colon which can turn ulcerative), degenerative joint disease, and skin disorders.

This abstract by Galland and Barrie concluded that "reducing fat and meat and ingesting soluble fiber, Bifidobacteria, Lactobacillus, and Bacillus laterosporus preparations contributed to an overall correction of intestinal dysbiosis," when the harmful bacteria outnumber the beneficial bacteria. [3]

In the past decade, researchers have discovered that parasites, including Candida albicans, have the ability to mutate. In 1985, microbiologist David R. Soll, Ph.D., reported in *Science* that Candida albicans, the major yeast pathogen in humans, is capable of changing to another form and then changing back again to its original shape. It has at least 17 variants! [4] This quick-change capability allows the fungus to elude the immune system and resist antifungal medications.

Nine years after the initial fungi-mutating information by Dr. Soll appeared, the same journal published a 33-page collection of eleven articles documenting how bacteria and fungi mutate to evade antibiotics and antifungal drugs. Basically, these organisms have devised several ways to save themselves from destruction via the following methods of mutation: 1. production of an efficient pump that ejects the antibiotics before they can harm the bacteria; 2. construction of a strong cell wall that prevents penetration by antibiotics; 3. manufacture of enzymes that destroy or inactivate antibiotics; 4. movement of parts of the bacteria DNA to another place, called gene jumping, which causes cells to take on different forms; and 5. development of substitute proteins not targeted by antibiotics. [5] Bacteria have become resistant to antibiotics because of their excessive use.

One frightening example of drug-resistant bacteria occurred in New York in 1992. Dr. Elizabeth Seaton, a 35-year-old neonatologist, pregnant with her second child, was just three days short of reaching full-term when she entered the hospital because of fever, abdominal cramping, and diarrhea. Thirty-five minutes after she entered the hospital, the residents realized the unborn baby was in serious trouble and the baby was born dead minutes later. Then the fight for the mother's life began, ending three days later when she also died. Some bacteria release toxins throughout the body, killing cells. This causes the circulatory system to fail and the body's vital organs to collapse. Despite the fact that Dr. Seaton was being cared for at a major university medical center, a valiant fight with three powerful antibiotic drugs, ampicillin, clindamycin, and gentamicin, were useless. [6] Mother and baby were victims of a bacterial strain of streptococcus which had developed a resistance to all forms of antibiotics.

If you get this type of infection, states Dr. Michael Cohen of the federal Center for Disease Control (CDC) and Prevention in Atlanta, "you are in the Almighty's hands." [7] Even the administrators at the federal CDC feel there is cause for alarm, especially for those whose immune systems have been compromised by severe and/or chronic illness.

Bacterial overgrowth also can cause contagious diseases, such as peptic ulcer. Previously this familiar malady affecting millions of people, or nearly one in ten adults, was believed to be caused by stress. However, a young, brash Australian medical doctor, Barry Marshall, proved it other-wise. [8, 9] It had previously been believed that harmful bacteria could not survive stomach acid. Dr. Marshall proved that this bacteria, Helicobacter, corkscrews through the mucus and settles just beyond the stomach lining. To insure survival, Helicobacter then coats itself with enzymes for protection from stomach acid. This bacteria is now believed to initially cause an infection in the stomach lining. This infection can then develop into an ulcer. If not treated, over a period of many years it can turn into stomach cancer. Patients afflicted with this disorder complain of digestive symptoms, such as a burning stomach pain which seems to intensify when the stomach is empty. Since eating relieves the pain, the patient eats frequently resulting in excess weight.

Along with fungus and bacteria, many people are plagued with parasitic worms. These parasites start out in the intestine, but can affect other tissues. Dr. James Jackson in the Department of Clinical Sciences at Wichita State University in Kansas agrees that "non-specific gastrointestinal symptoms and persistent diarrhea may indicate intestinal parasites." [10] Estimates of those suffering with parasites range from 18% to 75% of the general population. One reason for this wide range could be due to the accuracy of testing because of differential diagnostic techniques. A more specific test for the detection of parasites (based on a rectal swab) is used at the Center for the Improvement of Human Functioning in Wichita, Kansas. [11] This rectal swab test found a higher incidence of parasitic infestation than when stool samples only were sent to a laboratory. In 377 samples, the Center found 11.1% contained Entamoeba histolytica; 3.7% had Giardia Lamblia; 2.1% Ascariasis; and 6.9% Hookworm filariform.

Health care professionals such as Dr. Galland agree that a rectal swab is superior to a stool culture in diagnosing the presence of parasites. However, some feel that in obtaining the rectal swab it is important to obtain as much mucus as possible. [12] The probability of the presence of parasites is higher if there is a concentration of mucus in the stool. A sample containing more mucus and less stool demonstrates the existence of a greater number of parasites.

All types of parasites can cause problems for their hosts. Allergist and CRC expert William Crook, M.D., writes, "bacterial overgrowth in the small intestine in patients with giardiasis (infestation by parasitic Giardia) may contribute to malabsorption and nutritional deficiencies and may also promote the colonization of Candida albicans." [13] An overgrowth of bacteria may also cause chronic fatigue. He also states that elimination of giardiasis resulted in less fatigue in 70% of the 218 patients.

Where are we getting these parasites? They are spread through contaminated water and food, transmitted via sexual contact, and through contact with family members. Pets can be a another source. One instance of water contamination occurred in Milwaukee, Wisconsin in April of 1993. [14] The city's filtration system was overworked by a high level of runoff from farms and slaughterhouses. City water then became contaminated with the parasite worm called cryptosporidiosis. This caused thousands to become ill with diarrhea and other intestinal symptoms and even caused several deaths. Milwaukee is not the only city to have problems with their water. In 1984, the CDC investigated outbreaks in five other states. [15]

Researchers in a European study published in the American Society for Microbiology journal state they have found one avenue by which parasites are entering our food chain. This study showed that sewage sludge spread on farmland contained viable parasite eggs. In fact, each hectare (equal to 2.47 acres) studied showed 20,280,000 viable Taenia saginata parasitic eggs per nine metric tons of sewage sludge. The danger lies in sewage sludge spread over grazing or pasture land. [16] The cattle can be infected and this infection can in turn reach humans from insufficiently cooked meat. In order to kill parasites, the food temperature needs to reach 180 degrees Fahrenheit.

Health and massage therapist Stanley Weinberger conducted the first major nationwide survey of parasitic diseases. His survey revealed that one in every six people has one or more parasites living somewhere in his or her body. Weinberger states that if we eliminate parasites we are taking one of the most important steps to restore and maintain optimal health. [17]

Nutritional parasitic expert and author Ann Louise Gittleman, M.S., believes that parasitic worms are an underlying cause of disease. Since most people are loath to discuss such an indelicate subject, not many research dollars are devoted to finding a cure. While parasitic disease affects one hundred times as many people as cancer, $800 million is spent on cancer research and less than $1 million on parasitic disease research. In her clinic—which includes environmentally-oriented doctors and special diagnostic laboratories—an astounding three out of four patients tested positive for parasites. [18] Gittleman discovered that most people are carrying around four to five types of parasites of which Candida albicans is but one.

Gittleman noted that in her practice a wide variety of diseases like food and chemical allergies, diabetes, hypoglycemia, constipation, diarrhea, ulcers, tumors, depression, and even chronic fatigue disappeared after parasitic worms were cleared from the system and beneficial bacteria was restored to the gastrointestinal tract.

Gittleman relates her experiences in ridding the body of parasites:
In my practice I have obtained the best results using a combination of hydrated bentonite clay and powdered psyllium husks . . . Bentonite is said to absorb up to 180 times its own weight in bacteria, toxic debris, and even parasites . . . Psyllium acts like a broom to help eliminate stagnant waste in the gut. [19]

Psyllium is an intestinal cleanser. Bentonite absorbs the harmful toxins produced by fungi, bacteria, and worms and flushes them out of the body. The combination of these two products are a great aid in eliminating toxins from the intestinal tract.

Some researchers feel that the cause of parasitic mutation is the heavy use of antibiotics in farm animals (which appear on our dinner plate) and overprescription of antibiotics in humans. Often doctors prescribe antibiotics in response to insistent pleas from patients who demand an antibiotic for an illness that would be self-limiting and terminate without the use of antibiotics.

CRC patients, especially those who acquired this illness due to the intake of too many antibiotics, hope that those in medicine and agriculture will realize the dangers of overuse of antibiotics and prescribe them only when absolutely necessary.

Penicillin, the first antibiotic, came on the market in 1940 to fight infection caused by bacteria. Many other antibiotics followed and there are now 100 varieties on the market. Fifty years later, bacteria are becoming more resistant to drugs; common bacteria are able to defend themselves against previously-successful drug treatments. One of the common bacterium causes ear infections, which result in at least half of the 24 million annual office visits to pediatricians for earaches annually. [20]

Since parasites, fungi, bacteria, and worms are becoming resistant to drugs, and (more importantly) because prescription drugs may have harmful side effects, many alternative health care professionals are using non-toxic parasite therapy. Clearing the intestinal tract of parasites and keeping the body free of their return can be done with natural remedies including: caprylic acid (liquid form works best), psyllium, bentonite, friendly flora, Echinacea (an immune-boosting herb), vitamins and minerals, proper rest, food, and exercise.

Alternative health care professionals suggest that to rid the body of parasites one should clean out the gastrointestinal tract using natural therapeutic treatments and reimplant beneficial bacteria. Some therapists also recommend colonic irrigation, a gentle washing of the colon or large intestine combined with external massage. One must correct a diet which is high in sugar, refined carbohydrates, raw or undercooked beef, pork and fish, and fiber-depleted processed foods. Lack of fiber slows the peristaltic action resulting in constipation. This results in impacted fecal matter—a rich breeding ground for parasites and bacteria.

Part Two

Three-Prong Therapy Approach
Used in Study

Chapter Seven

Acupuncture and Candida Related Complex

This part of the book will discuss five areas: 1. acupuncture, how it works and how it can help heal those who have Candida Related Complex (CRC); 2. diet, modifications must be made for the CRC patient to improve; 3. treatment program, several products are mixed together for ingestion twice daily; 4. how the above three procedures help to rid the body of CRC when other procedures have previously failed; and 5. other natural therapies which also help those with CRC.

Acupuncture

Acupuncture has been used for thousands of years in China, so its effectiveness has been tested over and over again throughout the millennia. Recent research has validated acupuncture's effectiveness for many illnesses, including CRC, and a variety of symptoms affecting not only the physical, but the spiritual and mental health of patients.

The word acupuncture comes from the Latin words "acus," meaning needle, and "punctura," meaning to prick. Using needles to prick the skin at specific spots, practitioners are able to restore the proper balance of energy, what acupuncturists refer to as chi (pronounced "chee"). This treatment was little known in the United States until James Reston, a writer for the *New York Times*, had emergency surgery while in China in 1971 and experienced postoperative pain relief from acupuncture. [1] His subsequent writings about this experience aroused interest in acupuncture throughout the nation.

The saying "look to the old to discover the new" has inspired many current uses of acupuncture. Numerous texts describe a sophisticated system of study using acupuncture's energy meridian concept for treating human ailments. Through the study of the ancient writings, one discovers that as early as 2000 B.C. the early Chinese masters had a deep and thorough understanding of the laws of the universe, the origins of disease, and the life force which drives all living things.

Only recently have modern scientists come to understand the fact that invisible energy vibration and matter are not two separate phenomena, but are actually the same at their fundamental level; that is, matter can be converted to energy and vice versa. This modern finding by Western physicians is mentioned quite matter-of-factly in the *Nei Ching Su Wen*, a Chinese medical philosophy book written approximately five thousand years ago by a master named Huang Ti. [2] The text explains that there is an energy force, or chi, that circulates in meridians or channels throughout the body. The character and quality of this chi influences the functioning of different organs and systems in the body. This ancient book is available in English from the University of California Press.

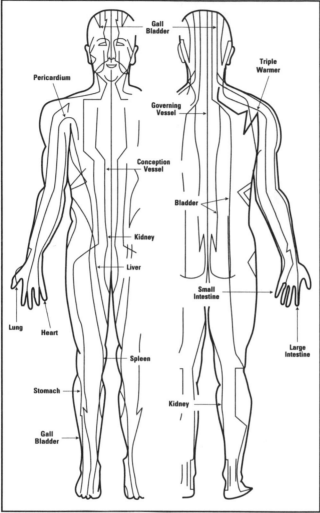

The major body meridians.

A medical dictionary gives this description of acupuncture: a modality developed in China for certain types of anesthesia and treatment of various disorders by insertion of fine stainless steel needles into specific areas of the body; it is thought to work through the body's autonomic nervous system. Also called neuronyxis. [3]

By analyzing neuronyxis, a synonym for acupuncture, we can learn more about acupuncture. The root word of neuronyxis, neuron, means:

The basic functional and anatomic unit of the nervous system, concerned with the conduction of impulses: structurally, it is the most complex cell of the body; the human nervous system contains about twenty-eight billion neurons. [4]

From the above, we can see that Chinese medicine falls into Western medicine's neurology department.

Meridians

The practice of acupuncture is based on the concept of an acupuncturist (through the use of needles) bringing back the needed balance in order to maintain or restore health. This is done by assessing the character and quality of the chi in the meridians through the twelve pulses felt in the radial side of the wrists, six in each wrist.

There are fourteen major meridians, each one named after the organ it controls. For example, the points in the lung meridian can be used to treat lung-related problems and the points in the kidney meridian

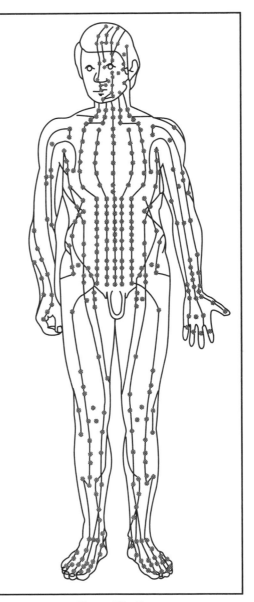

The meridian lines.

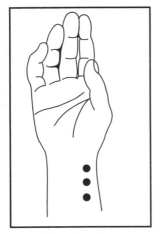

The meridian pulses.

can be used to treat kidney-related problems. Fifty-seven other secondary meridians complete the network. Energy points are located a few centimeters beneath the skin's surface along the course of the meridians.

One of the most interesting aspects of the Chinese system of healing is the correspondence between the major organ meridians and seemingly unrelated issues. For example, the kidneys are associated with the health of the bones and the lower back. A weakness in the kidneys often results in lower back pain and/or bone disease. One of acupuncture's basic principles is that any symptom or weakness is a reflection of an underlying imbalance or weakness of one or more of the major organs or channels.

In addition to the physical symptoms, specific psychological and emotional patterns are associated with the meridians and the organs they represent. Chinese medicine is credited with having the most sophisticated model of holism because, as ancient as this system of healing is, it holds that the mind, spirit, and body are an inseparable unit. What affects one element affects the other two as well.

The following comparison chart is an example of how Chinese medicine attributes harmful emotions to the imbalance or illness of organs.

WHICH EMOTIONS AFFECT WHICH ORGANS

Grief	Lungs, Large intestines
Worry, Brooding	Stomach, Spleen
Overexcitement, Joy	Heart, Small intestines
Fear, Insecurity	Kidneys, Urinary bladder
Anger, Frustration	Liver, Gallbladder

This chart shows that grief affects the lungs. For example, a recent widow can attest to the fact that when grief is intense, it is difficult to breathe; grief is affecting the lungs. Or when a worker has an argument with his employer, he feels a pain in his stomach; worry and brooding are affecting his stomach.

Another precept held by the ancient Chinese masters is the understanding that human beings are influenced by the seasons and the natural weather patterns. The masters observed that seasonal climates and varying daylight hours have a distinct effect on the meridians and predispose some people to certain diseases.

Today, scientists are learning just how and why we are affected by light. Some people suffer from Seasonal Affective Disorder (SAD) due to insufficient sunlight. An expert in the study of light, John Ott, explored the connection between exposure to light energy and cancer, and the effect of several lighting systems on the pineal and pituitary glands. [5] Ott's interest in light led him to the position of Director of the Environmental Health and Light Research Institute in Florida, where pioneering light research is being conducted.

Acupuncture assists the body's healing by helping organs return to a proper balance of energy, rather than being at a too high or yang (overactive) level, or a too low or yin (underactive) level (as is the case for many CRC patients). For example, the liver may not be getting enough energy or blood flow (underactive) or it may be getting too much energy and become inflamed (overactive).

Acupuncture also facilitates the body's ability to increase its resistance to allergens and to alleviate the many sensitivities from which patients suffer. As previously discussed, CRC patients experience sensitivities to various foods, molds, and scents. For some, this becomes debilitating. Unfortunately, the side effects of medications prescribed to alleviate the pain and inflammation can wreak further havoc in their already-weakened systems. It is in precisely this situation that acupuncture can provide relief. It is successful in alleviating pain without introducing toxic substances into a patient's already-hypersensitive body. Acupuncture works *with* (not against) the wounded person.

Methods of Acupuncture Stimulation

There are six methods used to influence energy flow: acupuncture needles; heated needles (procedure called moxibustion); vacuum (procedure called cupping); electrical stimulation; acupressure; or laser. When these points are stimulated, they effect a change in the chi and this produces predictable physiological changes.

Stimulating the acupuncture point by any of these six means sends a message to the brain (the hypothalamus) which is then interpreted and decoded. Messages are then sent to the body's defense mechanism through the autonomic nervous system. "This in turn enhances the natural healing process of the body to relieve pain and help cure the disease," states an Ohio physician Sung S. Kim in the *American Journal of Acupuncture*. [6]

Needling with acupuncture needles is the most common form of influencing energy flow. Using this method, the acupuncturist inserts a sterilized needle into the acupuncture point and sometimes twirls or pumps the needle to bring forth the energy. Usually the patient feels a slight pinprick and an electrical sensation as the tip of the needle connects with the energy point.

Moxibustion is the process of warming a needle to stimulate energy flow. "Moxa" is the Chinese name for herbal cones made of dried mug wort leaves, garlic, and ginger. In moxibustion, a small cone of moxa is placed around the head (or the end) of the needle. The moxa is not inserted into the skin. Modern methods use burning moxa discs placed around the base of the inserted needle. Moxibustion provides heat, which produces a stronger stimulation of chi or energy than by using the needle alone.

Cupping is another technique used to stimulate acupuncture points. The practitioner causes local congestion of blood by using a small cup, creating a vacuum by heat. Thus, cupping brings vital energy to a specific area. [7]

Electrical stimulation is another technique. Clamps connected to a wire are attached to the inserted acupuncture needle. A low-frequency current can thus be regulated by the acupuncturist, using nine-volt electronic equipment.

Acupressure is a non-invasive technique in which the acupuncturist applies stimulation to acupuncture points using finger pressure. Acupressure is another form of stimulation that can help relieve pain and restore health. For example, pressure in the wedge between the thumb and forefinger helps to relieve pain such as toothache or headache.

Because some of his patients have difficulty understanding how acupuncture works, Dr. Sung S. Kim tells his patients that it works like a computer:

> A computer recognizes the 'bit,' which is short for binary digit. It can have only two possible values—0 or 1. All data (letters, numerals, symbols) handled by computers are digitalized and expressed as combinations of bits—0s and 1s. Another way of expressing this is (-) or (+), negative or positive, or yin and yang.
>
> However complex the computer appears to be, it boils down to a byte, which contains eight bits of information. A bit is to a byte what a

letter is to a word—the tiniest unit of memory. It then becomes apparent that inserting a needle into an acupuncture point is like typing on a computer keyboard. Signals given at a local point will be transmitted to the hypothalamus instantly, through different routes. [8]

In today's computer-literate culture, individuals can easily use this computer analogy to more readily understand acupuncture's healing technique.

There are several theories which are the basis of the ideas behind acupuncture. Two of the more basic ones are the Yin/Yang Theory and the Theory of Five Elements.

Yin/Yang Theory

The Yin/Yang Theory is used to understand and analyze body processes. It represents a combination of unified opposites and a constant movement of energy between these two opposites. If the flow of energy is obstructed or overactive, then the body falls ill. One opposite does not exist without the other and each is constantly changing into its opposite—a constant flow of energy or chi. This theory relates to the previously mentioned concept regarding the constant intermingling of matter and energy. In the context of yin/yang, matter is yin and energy is yang. Other yin/yang examples are cold and hot, weak and strong, female and male, night and day, hypofunction and hyperfunction, and rest and activity. Acupuncturists correct imbalances and encourage the chi to flow properly again.

Five Elements Theory

The Five Elements Theory is used to explain the relationship between people and their environment. The five elements represent five basic energies in nature, which are symbolized by five substances in nature: wood, fire, earth, metal, and water. Each element corresponds to a specific organ in the body, season, emotion, psychic or mental activity, bodily tissue, and sound. For example, wood represents the liver, spring, anger, planning, tendons, and shouting. This theory evolved from observation of the changing patterns in nature and is an elaboration of the Yin/Yang theory.

The five elements are like phases in a cycle of gradation from yin to yang. Water has the most yin and fire has the most yang. Metal and wood are transition points between the two extremes and earth is considered in the middle. The idea behind these phases is that they are all mutually dependent on each other. Each phase or element generates the next. Also, each element is controlled, or controls another element. For example, wood creates fire, is controlled by metal, and controls earth. Translated to the organ/meridian correspondences, it follows that the liver generates the heart, is controlled by the lungs, and controls the spleen. Using the principles of the Five Elements Theory allows the practitioner to understand the progress of a disease and to predict its prognosis.

The main principle of acupuncture treatment is to enhance the quality of the chi or energy. Chi circulates within the meridians and can be influenced by needling the acupuncture points. Each point produces certain predictable physiological changes. The two main bases for the selection of points in acupuncture treatment is the pattern of yin and yang found in the patient and the status of the five elements of wood, fire, earth, metal, and water as portrayed in the patient's pulses. This system considers the influence of the environment, climate, diet, activity, and emotions. It sees symptoms as a reflection of an underlying imbalance in chi or energy.

The beauty of Chinese medicine is that it is holistic. It is a very natural approach, does not involve the use of chemicals, and is relatively inexpensive. It is a system that treats the cause of the illness, not just the symptoms.

Patients usually need a series of acupuncture treatments spaced at regular intervals. The number of treatments depends on the severity and chronicity of the illness. Acupuncture offers an alternative to chemical drugs and surgery. It works hand in hand with other holistic systems of healing, such as natural immune boosters, nutrition, and massage. Some patients may experience minor short-term effects from an acupuncture treatment for several days following the treatment, such as aching, a slight hematoma (black and blue mark), or a rash. However, acupuncture seldom has harmful effects. Drugs, on the other hand, generally do have side effects that range from minor to major, and that are sometimes even fatal.

Patterns of illness are pieced together by the skilled acupuncture practitioner based on the symptoms as expressed by the patient, the findings from the pulse, and the color and coating of the tongue. In both Eastern and Western medicine, the tongue is used to evaluate diseases. The body of the tongue is examined for color. Normal color is a nice pink. A too-pale or too-red tongue indicates an imbalance. A white coating signifies a cold or a deficiency syndrome. A yellow coating signifies excess heat in the body; heat may be indicative of infection or inflammation.

These illnesses may follow a certain pattern that may be called yin-yang, cold-heat, dryness-dampness (dehydration-fluid retention), or external-internal. For example, a patient who complains of low energy, fatigue, a tendency to feel cold, and has dry, itchy skin can be said to have a deficiency/weakness pattern. This is a "yin" condition, with not enough chi circulating in the channels. This situation would be the opposite of a "yang" pattern of jitteriness or jumpiness—the patient is very active, irritable, looks red in the face, and probably has high blood pressure. Acupuncture treatments can strengthen a channel that has weak chi or calm a channel that has excess chi.

For a more in-depth look at acupuncture from the patient's perspective, the reader is referred to the book entitled *Acupuncture—A Patient's Guide* by Dr. Paul Marcus. [9] This book explains what can be expected of acupuncture, which conditions it will benefit, where to go for acupuncture, and is a good general guidebook for the patient.

Acupuncture as a Healing Technique for CRC

In the study at the East West Clinic, acupuncture is used as one of the three foundation blocks of CRC treatment. The other two are diet with a nutritional supplement program and the use of fungicides and colon cleansers.

Acupuncture is used for specific symptoms which may vary from CRC patient to CRC patient. One patient may have bronchitis and Candida pneumonia as the primary symptoms, while another may have severe anxiety, depression, fatigue, and a low energy level. The acupuncturist can use different combinations of points to address the various manifestations of the disease.

Acupuncture, CRC, and Food Cravings

There are many acupuncture points in the auricle of the ears that are needled to help the whole body function properly. Auricle refers to the visible exterior portion of the ear. As early as 1975, two physicians on opposite sides of the United States reported on their success using auricular medicine to treat obesity: Lester L. Sacks, M.D., in California, and Robert M. Giller, M.D., in New York. [10, 11] Four years later, a Midwest medical doctor, Evelyn Lee Sun, reported that acupressure on the auricle was also effective in weight reduction. [12] Acupressure is the process of applying finger pressure to the acupuncture points in the ear without piercing the skin with needles.

Then in 1984, the *Chinese Acupuncture & Moxibustion Journal* cited yet another study using auricular therapy in weight reduction. [13] Acupuncture's effectiveness in this area is so remarkable that food craving is one of the first CRC symptoms to be controlled.

Acupuncture, CRC, and Inflammations

Acupuncture treatments can raise the body's defensive energy, clear congestions, reduce inflammations, and increase circulation. CRC patients often complain of low energy, infections, and cold extremities. As noted by a group of researchers headed by Dr. Y. M. Sin at London's St. Bartholomew's Hospital in 1983, acupuncture is clinically effective in treating acute and chronic inflammatory disease. [14] Acupuncture can release endorphins (pain-relieving substances) and reduce inflammation.

Furthermore, acupuncture has been shown to halt disease. A year later Dr. Sin reported on another study on acupuncture and inflammation, concluding that "acupuncture stimulation not only gives good symptomatic relief in inflammatory disease but also actually suppresses the underlying progress of the disease." [15] The benefits of acupuncture in fighting disease are varied and multiple points are used to bring predictable outcomes for the variety and multiplicity of CRC symptoms.

Anti-inflammatory drugs are successful in treating chronic irritation, infection, or injury, but the long-term effects of these drugs are unknown. At least one illness, Cushing's disease, is actually caused by corticosteroids, a common anti-inflammatory drug. With illnesses such as rheumatoid arthritis, which has traditionally been treated by prolonged doses of anti-inflammatory drugs, patients can use acupuncture therapy as an excellent alternative, eliminating further exposure to the damaging effects of drugs. [16] Acupuncture is especially necessary if the patient is exhibiting severe side effects to drug therapy.

Acupuncture, CRC, and Pain

Acupuncture treatments can be used on local areas to reduce swelling and pain. As an example, some CRC patients experience recurring headaches, muscle weakness, or persistent coughing. Acupuncture can also be used systemically to balance organ dysfunctions brought on by CRC, and generally stimulate the body's ability to heal naturally.

Acupuncture, CRC, and Immune Dysfunction

CRC is an immunodeficiency disease, meaning it results from a weakened immune system. CRC patients are unable to contain the growth of the fungi within. Research using both animal and human subjects has documented the effectiveness of acupuncture in strengthening the immune system. Results published in four separate articles in the *American Journal of Acupuncture* cite the following benefits of acupuncture to the immune system: 1. increased granulation of mast cells; 2. initially decreased leukocyte count after thirty minutes, and an increase of as much as 168% by the third hour; 3. increased bactericidal power of plasma (increase in the ability of the blood to kill harmful bacteria); and 4. increased antibody production, as well as many other benefits. [17, 18, 19, 20]

Early intervention with acupuncture, Chinese herbal medicine, lifestyle changes, diet and stress reduction are all helpful in immunodeficiency diseases. "Acupuncture works on a deep spiritual level as well as on a physical energetic level . . . Changes in the emotional or spiritual state often stimulate changes in the physical body." [19] This is familiar to students of psychology who know that a very high percentage of physical illnesses are psychosomatic in origin.

A Russian researcher, Peter Pugach, reported on his work, stating that "manipulation of biologically active points of the body produce stimulating and regulating effects on the immune system of the organism." [20] Throughout the world, especially in Asia and Europe, scientists are finding that acupuncture is an effective treatment modality.

Acupuncture, CRC, and Itching

In some CRC patients the overgrowth of fungus manifests itself on the skin. Mycosis fungoides (a skin disease caused by a fungus) produces ulceration with oozing, often the result of scratching, especially on the neck and back. [21] The symptoms are itching, scratching, and dark red and rough scaly skin anywhere even in the hands and feet. Twenty acupuncture treatments were effective in eliminating the disease from one patient, as reported by Chinese physician He Hon Lao in the *American Journal of Acupuncture*. Acupuncture successfully stopped the itching and the resultant painful manifestations. I have personally observed the effectiveness of acupuncture for skin problems repeatedly in my own clinical practice.

Acceptance of Acupuncture

Acupuncture is being accepted by general practitioners around the world. A study of 370 doctors in Auckland, New Zealand, were surveyed; 249 responded. Seventy-five of the respondents (or 30%) stated they practiced alternative medicine. Of those alternative methods, acupuncture was cited as the most common therapy. One hundred and seventy-one doctors (or 69%) said they referred patients to some type of alternative medicine. Only 56 (or 32.7%) of the 171 doctors who said they referred patients to alternative medicine felt it was necessary that the person performing the procedure had any Western medical background. One hundred and seventy-six of the doctors who practiced alternative medicine (71%) used acupuncture themselves, and 89.5% of doctors who referred patients to alternative treatment listed acupuncture as possible therapy for their patients. The same study reported that acupuncture ranked third in the

United Kingdom as the most common therapy used by alternative practitioners. "The survey demonstrates that alternative practices are now an integral part of primary health care." [22]

Additionally, 1,000 U.S. pharmacists and 750 British pharmacists were surveyed on their feelings regarding alternative health approaches. Only 19.7% in the U.S. responded, though 63% of pharmacists in Britain did. Of those responding, 83.8% from the U.S. and 91% from Britain felt that acupuncture was the most useful alternative health approach. [23]

Acupuncture is Cost Effective

While some traditional medical personnel are using acupuncture themselves or are referring patients to acupuncturists, a study in *Neurology* reported that stroke patients recovered more quickly when acupuncture was added to their treatment. This resulted in substantial monetary savings.

This Swedish study followed 78 patients in Sweden. These patients were divided into two groups. One group received acupuncture treatments, (labeled "sensory stimulation" in the journal) and the second group received no sensory stimulation. The study concluded that patients whose treatment included acupuncture improved more quickly than the control group. Improvements were measured in the areas of motor function, balance, activities of daily living, and quality of life. The study also compared time needed for hospitalized rehabilitation in the two groups. After a year, only 9% of those receiving acupuncture were still hospitalized as compared to the control group where 30% remained hospitalized. The financial consequences demonstrated a hospital-cost savings of $26,000 per patient. [24] Thus, in addition to being an effective treatment modality, acupuncture can be a substantial cost-saving measure.

Conclusion

In summary, acupuncture has been used successfully for thousands of years in the Far East and is gaining acceptance among Western medical personnel. Stimulation of specific acupuncture body points can have a positive effect elsewhere in the body. Acupuncture can help CRC patients with their overall healing, food cravings, pain, and severe itching by stimulating the immune system. It is also being accepted as a valid complementary, and sometimes alternative, therapy to Western medicine. When acupuncture is used in conjunction with traditional treatment, recovery time is quicker than without acupuncture. In addition, there is a considerable financial savings, because recovery time is shortened.

Case Study Four

21-Year-Old Female With Panic Attacks, Agoraphobia

My name is Mary, and I am 21-year-old single student. My problems started in December, 1993, when I began to experience panic attacks as well as symptoms of agoraphobia (abnormal fear of open spaces). I did not know what was happening to me. I only knew I was very nervous and the physicians I consulted did not seem to know what was wrong with me. I finally found a psychiatrist willing to see me and she prescribed some anti-anxiety drugs which helped alleviate my severe anxiety. I also began to see a psychologist for psychotherapy sessions, but my symptoms persisted and, in fact, got progressively worse.

My mother is a nurse and suggested I see Colet Lahoz, an acupuncturist who is also a nurse with professional training in traditional Chinese medicine. I felt so sick, I was willing to try anything. My symptoms consisted of a racing heart rate, frequent bouts of diarrhea, insomnia, nausea, and a pervasive fearful feeling. I was terrified at being left alone and of driving, especially by myself. When I had my first session, she told me in no uncertain terms that I would get better. This was very reassuring.

At first I had acupuncture treatments twice a week and, as I got better, only once a week. I began to feel more relaxed and less scared. My other physical symptoms began to disappear as well. After the first month of acupuncture therapy, I was finally able to stand being alone without panicking and I sensed an overall feeling of wellness. At the suggestion of my acupuncturist, I started using relaxation and self-healing tapes. I also practiced yoga and received therapeutic massage once a week.

After a month or two, I was able to function somewhat normally again, but was still not feeling well. Some new symptoms I noticed included a red rash on my back, feelings of "spaciness," exhaustion, dizziness, and depression. I was also still experiencing a loss of appetite, insomnia, and anxiety. Though I was no longer experiencing terrifying panic attacks, I was still not feeling very well.

My acupuncturist suggested that I take the "Rate Yourself Questionnaire" by Dr. Trowbridge to rule out systemic Candida infection. I did and tested positive. She then suggested I try the colon cleansing program and go on a yeast-free, sugar-free diet. I did not pursue her suggestion at first because I wanted to wait and see if the symptoms would go away on their own.

The symptoms persisted another month and that is when I decided it was time to go with her advice. I gave up all foods containing yeast or sugar. After just a few days, I started to feel better and some of the dizziness disappeared. I no longer felt like the world was spinning around me. My mood also improved a little and I was less irritable. Every time I went off the diet, the symptoms would return. I went out drinking one night and ate food with a lot of sugar. The following morning I felt especially dizzy, anxious, and irritable. The rash on my back (which had lightened up) became larger and redder. I had a long history with this rash. It covered the whole extent of my back and a dermatologist I had consulted at one time thought part of it was acne, but did not know what the other red spots were. Now I know that the acupuncturist was right when she said they were fungi or yeast related.

I had initially thought that I did not need the colon cleansing part of the program, that my depression was just situational and this phase would pass. However, since the depression and all the other symptoms were not completely going away, I decided to do the colon cleansing program as well. I started the combination of Caprol, bentonite, psyllium, and acidophilus the next day. In just a few days, my mood improved tremendously. I was actually feeling happy at times. I could once again sleep through the night without waking up at two in the morning and staying restless for hours. My depression started lifting and my anxiety significantly decreased. The rash covering my back was quickly drying up.

It has been a long road to recovery for me. I had been thinking what episode in my life might have brought this on. I have not taken antibiotics or cortisone therapy, but I was on birth control pills for three years because of an irregular menstrual cycle. According to my acupuncture therapist, this alone was sufficient to predispose me to develop candidiasis. My experience with alternative healing methods has certainly been very impressive. I would encourage anyone suffering from similar health concerns to try these methods as well, especially when Western medicine is not able to diagnose or treat the problem, as in my own case.

—Mary Bajari, Annandale, Minnesota

Chapter Eight

Diet and Candida Related Complex

Diet, the second component of the treatment protocol for Candida Related Complex (CRC), plays an enormous part in the recovery process. In addition to a healthy diet, CRC patients need additional nutritional support in the form of supplemental vitamins and minerals. This chapter will examine proper food combining, the many benefits of wholesome, fresh vegetables, the degree to which our food has become tainted with poisonous substances, and how proper food preparation can negate these harmful effects.

Strict adherence to the diet is required for success in therapy. It is as important as the other aspects: acupuncture, fungicides, colon cleansers, and a nutritional supplementation program.

Results of a Poor Diet

The diet of the average North American consists of food that is over-processed, low in fiber, and high in refined sugar. We also consume large amounts of red meat, dairy products, and wheat. According to a 1977 *Journal of the American Medical Association* article, this diet results in fewer "friendly bacteria" in the intestinal tract. [1] Furthermore, many of us eat too much, too often, and we mix too many different types of food in the same meal.

These and other factors provide an excellent breeding ground for Candida albicans. The unhealthy American diet causes a thick coat of mucus and impacted food residue to form on the walls of the large intestine, which prevents absorption of nutrients while also allowing absorption of toxins—the byproducts of fungi. The result is malnourishment. Bernard Jensen, D.C., in his book *Tissue Cleansing through Bowel Management*, identifies disease as actually beginning in the bowel. [2] Not only does this encrusted matter in the large intestine contribute to several dysfunctions of the colon, it also directly causes general poor health.

Candida albicans, normally inhabiting colons of even healthy individuals, really prefer to exist in a polluted colon because they thrive in an environment which is short of oxygen and putrid. When CRC patients clean out their colons, the fungi retreat to their former harmless state.

Internist Leo Galland, who is knowledgeable about both nutrition and CRC, reports that there are specific nutritional deficiencies generally found in CRC patients. [3] These include: vitamin B6, magnesium, abnormal metabolism of essential fatty acids, iron, vitamin A, and zinc. He has also discovered that about 66% of CRC patients have mitral valve prolapse (MVP). The mitral valve is located in the left side of the heart and links the upper chamber to the ventricle (cavity) below. Magnesium deficiency is suspected as a cause of MVP. The symptoms of MVP include chest pain, palpitation, fatigue, dizziness, poor exercise tolerance, anxiety, and hyperventilation.

Necessary Nutritional Tips

For those with CRC, dietary modifications are essential for successful recovery, states a *Candida* newsletter. [4] It is recommended that these patients adopt the following nutritional steps:

Changes for Eradicating CRC

- Eliminate refined sugars and refined, bleached, chemically-treated flour;
- Eliminate meats treated with synthetic hormones or chemicals;
- Eliminate hydrogenated fats (such as those that exist in peanut butter, baked goods, and margarine);
- Reduce fats (use those rich in flaxseed oil, Omega-3, fish and olive oils);
- Eat fresh and raw vegetables (comprising 40% of food consumed), fruit (30%), complex carbohydrates (20%), and protein (10%);
- Eat nothing unless it will spoil or rot, but eat it before it does so. At the grocery store, shop at the outer fringes of the building, avoiding canned and packaged products. Exercise regularly. Eliminate colon toxicity.

In addition to modifying the diet, CRC patients are advised to exercise and clean the colon where fungi proliferate and pollute.

It is understandable that patients find this change to be difficult at first. Many even resist the idea of beginning treatment if a diet modification is required because they doubt their ability to stick to a strict regimen. Most people eventually agree to try it because they are so tired of being sick that they are willing to try anything. In the end, they become convinced of the value of staying with the recommended diet, because they begin to feel well after many months (or even years) of being sick.

One consoling aspect about the anti-CRC diet is that it is temporary. Many patients need to be on a strict diet for only a few months while they are eliminating fungi from their system. They need to persevere until they are rid of the discomforts they suffer. The time required will vary from person to person. For the individuals in the CRC study at the East West Clinic, the symptoms disappeared, on the average, in two months. This average time is for the person who had been sick for a short time, has adhered to the anti-CRC diet, has taken the anti-fungal supplements, and has received acupuncture treatments.

Some practitioners feel that recovery takes one month for each year the patient has been sick. Others feel one should begin counting the months after an initial three month period, then add a month for every year of illness.

Most participants in our study, however, stayed with a less strict variation of the diet even after their condition had stabilized. They developed a taste for healthier foods and found a modified diet (more vegetables and no binging on sugar) to be a way to stay healthier and continue feeling well. Additionally, most found that their cravings for inappropriate foods had greatly lessened or ceased. They also discovered that if they overindulged in sugar or yeast, they experienced a return of familiar CRC symptoms.

Vitamins, a Nutritional Support

Vitamins (Latin "vita" and "mins" literally meaning life's necessity) have only recently been discovered; the word itself was coined in the year 1911. It wasn't until late in the 1800s that scientists became interested in the relationship between food and disease. Scientists then discovered that vitamin deficiencies can cause disease (i.e. vitamin D deficiency causes rickets) and vitamin sufficiencies can prevent disease (i.e. vitamin C sufficiency prevents scurvy).

Most of the work to be done in clearing the body of fungi is accomplished by the immune system. A sufficient vitamin supply strengthens the immune system. Unfortunately, CRC-afflicted individuals are often vitamin-depleted.

The general population has begun to realize the need for certain vitamins. In 1992-93, purchases of vitamin E rose by 39% over the previous two-year period. [5] Vitamin E has been found to reduce the risk of heart disease and can be found in wheat germ and nuts. At the same time, purchases of vitamin A rose by 31%. Vitamin A has been found to help prevent cancer. Among other foods, it is found in yellow vegetables—a food that CRC patients should consume.

Minerals, Another Nutritional Support

CRC patients also need to supplement their diet with minerals. Minerals, the spark plug of life, are involved in almost all enzyme reactions. An enzyme is a protein—secreted by a healthy body—that promotes a chemical change in other substances, while it remains unchanged.

Mineral imbalances can lead to metabolic dysfunction. Proper metabolic function is a chemical process which takes place in living tissue and is necessary for the maintenance of a living organism. A mineral imbalance will cause a significant disruption of this important function. For example, if people are deficient in iron, they may be anemic and lack energy. (Iron is naturally found in many nutritious foods including lean meat, shellfish, leafy green vegetables, and whole grain cereals.) Or if people are deficient in zinc, they may experience brittle hair and nails, prolonged wound healing, or painful joints. (Zinc is naturally found in bran, liver, and seafood.) Likewise, a chromium deficiency often causes sugar cravings, a common complaint of CRC patients.

At the East West Clinic, vitamins and minerals are tailored to the patients' needs. KM (a Matol product) is an effective herbal supplement that increases energy levels and detoxifies the system. Antioxidants like coenzyme Q10, Pycnogenol, Cat's Claw, Vitamins C and E, Beta Carotene, etc. are also recommended to boost the immune system. Garlic and grapefruit seed extract are used alternately with Caprol to eliminate mutating forms of fungi that become resistant to Caprol.

Nutritional vitamin and mineral supplemental needs will vary for each individual, depending upon age, medical condition, sex, and personal habits.

To evaluate one's need for specific vitamins or minerals, the CRC patient may wish to research this topic further. Hair analysis has proven to be 90% effective in evaluating deficiencies or excesses. Following a hair analysis, the laboratory will recommend any needed nutritional supplements.

Food Combining

Because most CRC patients have difficulty digesting foods, information about which foods can be combined at the same meal (without causing indigestion) is helpful. Dr. Herbert M. Shelton (1895-1985) first wrote about food combining in 1951. He suggested that eating foods in proper combination improves digestion, conserves the body's energy, maintains normal weight, increases nutrient availability, maintains blood alkalinity, decreases acid-forming toxins, and helps to eliminate gas and diarrhea.

When eating more than one type of food at a time, the body stimulates both acid and alkaline enzymes. [6] Protein digestion, for example, needs a highly acid medium for digestion, whereas carbohydrates and starches require an alkaline medium. If both of these types of foods are ingested at the same meal, the two enzymes interfere with each other and thus with the digestive process. This interference causes food to move along the digestive tract undigested, wasting valuable vitamins and minerals.

The following are some food-combining tips. Avoid eating carbohydrates with fruits, proteins with carbohydrates, two proteins at the same meal, fats with protein, and fruits with proteins and starches. Consume one starch per meal, fruit only with lettuce and celery, salads with proteins or starches, and melons alone.

Learning and using proper food combining techniques will maximize the amount of nutritional vitamins and minerals absorbed (necessary in the fight against CRC) as well as alleviate indigestion and intestinal problems. A book by Dennis Nelson, *Food Combining Simplified*, is a recommended source of information on food combining.

Vegetables

As previously noted, vegetable intake is necessary for a healthy body and CRC patients generally have a poor track record in eating enough of this food group. This could be a contributing factor in the overgrowth of Candida albicans in the first place. Fungi are opportunistic organisms. CRC patients are in a weakened condition, which allows the fungi to multiply and causes the already-impaired CRC patient to weaken further. It may surprise some individuals that vegetables, properly prepared, are delicious! It does not take a famous chef to create an appetizing vegetable dish and some experimentation in the kitchen will reveal which herbs and spices titillate your taste buds.

A series of articles in *Newsweek* touted the advantages of vegetables, calling them "the really healthful stuff." [7] The article goes on to state that, "vegetables contain compounds called phytochemicals that seem to reduce the risk of cancer . . . these new compounds offer the next great hope for health." Additionally, the article stated that phytochemicals are the "new frontier in cancer-prevention research" and are easily found in a variety of vegetables. The article also states that the National Cancer Institute has launched a multimillion-dollar research project to discover more about these phytochemicals derived from whole foods, especially vegetables and fruits.

Here is how cancer begins. A cancer-causing molecule invades a cell in our blood. This cancer-causing molecule can come from food, drink, air, or smoke. Vegetables can thwart cancer. For example, within only a few hours of consumption, broccoli's cancer-fighting phytochemicals enter the bloodstream. When they reach the cell with the cancer-causing molecule, they activate a group of proteins called Phase 2 Enzymes. The enzymes go to work attaching the carcinogen molecule to a healthy molecule which then pushes it out of the cell and into the bloodstream, where it is eliminated from the body. [8] This is an example of why we need to eat our vegetables!

Americans have reason for concern about colon cancer. In 1993, colon and rectal cancer ranked the second most common type of cancer for women (after breast cancer) and the third most common for men (after prostate and lung cancer). [9]

Food Preparation

The manner of food preparation affects the nutritional value of the food. It is best to eat vegetables and fruits as close to their raw, uncooked state as possible because foods in this state contain all their enzymes intact. Enzymes convert food into vital molecular structures which pass through the intestinal wall into the bloodstream, providing the body with necessary nourishment. There are three major groups of enzymes: metabolic enzymes, which work in blood, tissue, and organs; digestive enzymes, which help digest food so that it can be utilized by the body; and food enzymes, which come from raw food.

It is important to eat whole foods, such as vegetables and fruits. Even as recently as April 1994, scientists admitted that they have not yet identified all the valuable compounds existing in whole foods. [10] Since we can't get whole foods the easy way—by popping a vitamin pill—we need to go straight to the source: Nature's bounty.

There is one ominous note, however, regarding toxin-polluted vegetables. A 2,000-page 1994 Environmental Protection Agency report stated that toxins in our food are our most serious health hazard. The report states that dioxin, PCBs, and furans (by-products of incinerating chlorine-based chemicals) emit harmful chemicals which fall to earth and enter the food chain through animal fat, milk, eggs, and fish. [11] A landslide of new data on the toxic effects of these chemicals, especially dioxin, led the EPA to order an extensive three-year review.

A doctor with an oriental medical degree, Matt Van Benschoten, writing in the *American Journal of Acupuncture*, reported that he also found our food to be contaminated. He writes:

> Most animal products and produce are found to contain significant amounts of pesticide and/or antibiotic residues. The bioaccumulation of these toxins impairs the function of the immune, neurological, endocrine, and digestive systems, and appears to play a significant role for large numbers of patients with chronic relapsing infectious (CRC) and neurohormonal syndromes. [12]

Dr. Van Benschoten urges readers to buy only organically-grown produce and to eliminate dairy products from their diet, as these products appear to have the highest levels of toxic contamination.

Because of these environmental pollutants, appropriate steps must be taken in the preparation of food. Hazel R. Parcells, D.C., N.D., Ph.D., a researcher specializing in the field of energy and nutrition, advocates a procedure to eliminate all sprays, bacteria, fungus, and metallics from food. She suggests using a half teaspoon of Clorox to one gallon of water to create a bath in which to place fruits and vegetables for the following length of time:

PURIFYING SOAK BATH

thawed meat & fish, per pound*	5-10 minutes
thin-skinned fruits & vegetables	10 minutes
heavy-skinned fruits & root vegetables	15-30 minutes
eggs	20-30 minutes
apples & potatoes	30 minutes

*do not soak ground meat

Dr. Parcells recommends making a fresh batch of liquid bath mixture for each food group. Instead of Clorox, Basic H, a product of Shaklee Corporation, may also be used in the same proportion described above. Liquid organic concentrate by Amway is another product used for this purpose. Washing fruits and vegetables in this manner will make them healthy for the body; they will also stay fresher longer. Flavors will be greatly enhanced and harmful substances will be removed.

Snacks

Often CRC patients will become suddenly and overwhelmingly hungry. It is most helpful to have healthy, quick foods ready for instant consumption. If quick foods are not readily available, the CRC patient will be strongly tempted to snack on the wrong foods.

Recipes

Libraries and bookstores are excellent sources of cookbooks with healthy, sugar-free recipes. For example, *The Yeast Connection Cookbook* by William Crook, M.D. and Marjorie Hurt Jones and *The Candida Control Cookbook* by Gail Burton are good resources.

Foods to Avoid

Certain foods must be avoided when the CRC sufferer is ridding the body of fungi.

- Sugar, in all forms, including: very ripe fruits (the sugar in fruits also feeds the Candida and it is advisable to limit fruits during the first three months), desserts, cookies, pies, ice cream, candy, chocolates, white and brown sugar, honey, molasses, syrups, and sweetened soft drinks. Ice cream, besides being high in sugar and dairy, contains many harmful additives such as emulsifiers, thickening agents, and dyes. Polysorbate, an emulsifier used in making ice cream has been associated with the contaminant dioxane, know to cause cancer in animals. [13]

Refined, white sugar is the single most offending substance in regard to CRC. Yet, each U.S. citizen consumes an average of 72 pounds per year.

NutraSweet is to be avoided as well, because it feeds Candida albicans. A good alternative is vegetable glycerine or stevia, a natural sweetener from Paraguay, and natural juices after the initial stage (the first three months) of the anti-Candida program.

- Alcoholic beverages (Each shot of alcohol contains seven teaspoonfuls of sugar)
- Fermented products (vinegar, soy sauce, condiments such as sugar-laden catsup, mayonnaise, mustard, and salsas)
- Pickled foods (beets, pickles, relish, sauerkraut, and herring)
- Cured or processed meats (hot dogs, bacon, and luncheon meat)
- Mushrooms, all of which are a form of fungi
- Black tea
- Coffee, both regular and decaffeinated
- Yeast-containing products such as breads, crackers, etc. Some vitamins also contain yeast.
- Dairy products cause mucus to form in the intestines and encourage fungal overgrowth. Additionally, milk has been linked to various illnesses, including arthritis and heart disease. [15]

Foods to Limit
- Complex carbohydrates are restricted to 80 to 100 grams per day because they provide a good breeding ground for the yeast.

Foods to Include
Many of these items are sold in the "health food" section of the grocery store or in health food stores. Remember to read labels carefully.

- Lemon for its cleansing properties
- Garlic for its anti-fungal properties
- Raw onion for its natural antibiotic effect
- Beverages

Water, bottled spring water. Find a water source free of harmful additives. Chlorine destroys beneficial flora in gut. Fluoride causes cancer.

Herbal tea

Coffee substitutes

Unsweetened fruit juice (in small amounts) diluted with some water may be tolerated by some individuals and yet may cause a worsening of symptoms in others.

R.W. Knudsens Family Juices, bottled or in juice boxes.

Santa Cruz Natural organic Juices, bottled. These juices are organic. There are other brands that come without sugar but some have preservatives.

Some Dole and Seneca juices have no sugar added but may need to be diluted. Tree Top no-sugar-added frozen juices.

Freeze fresh, squeezed juice for a cool treat

The use of regular or decaffeinated coffee is not encouraged.

- Fresh fruits if not very ripe. Some people react even to the sugar contained in fruits.

  The sugar content is higher in very ripe fruit, so fruits that are semi-ripe are preferred

  Pears, apples, nectarines, peaches, etc.

  Dole canned pineapple in its natural juice

  Unsweetened banana chips

- Proteins

  Fresh, organically-grown meats and poultry are preferred, as they are not treated with antibiotics—sometimes called range chickens because these chickens are usually allowed free range to roam.

- Breads and crackers

  Any bread or cracker that is unleavened or baked without yeast is acceptable. French Meadows baked goods are often baked without yeast.

  Carr's Table Water Crackers with Sesame Seeds

  Nabisco Triscuit whole-wheat wafers

  Hain rice cakes

  Wasa Sesame Rye Crisp bread

  RYVTA Whole Grain Crisp bread

  Ralston Purina Natural Rye Krisp

  Guiltless Gourmet tortilla chips

  Corn tortillas (some of these flat breads have yeast)

  Whole grain muffins and biscuits

  Lefse

  Dimplflier yeast-free rye bread

  Essene Bread

  Whole-wheat Matzoh

  Whole grain pasta or pancakes

  Whole-wheat tortillas

  Rye Crisp

  Old Dutch Corn Chips

- Cereals

  Rolled Oats

- Cooked whole grain cereals are preferred such as millet, brown rice, whole wheat, and buckwheat.

  Some quick-cooking products include Oatmeal, Oat Bran, Roman Meal, Cream of Rye, and Seven Grain Cereal.

  Nature's Path Miller Rice Oatbran Flakes

  Erewon Whole Grain Crispy Brown Rice (Like Rice Krispies, they "snap, crackle and pop.")

  Kolln Oat Bran Crunch European High Fiber Cereal

  Kolln Crispy Oats European High Fiber Cereal

  Shredded Wheat

Buttermilk Biscuits
- Dairy
  Only plain yogurt or plain low-fat yogurt has no sugar.
  Plain Kefir
  Buttermilk
  Crispy crackers and triscuits are good dipped in yogurt. Mix yogurt with cut-up fresh semi-ripe fruit for a refreshing dessert or snack.
- Fats
  Butter
  Vegetable oils
- Cookies and desserts
  Golden Batch Sugar-Free Creme Wafers (cookies found in the diabetic or dietetic section of the grocery store)
- Nuts and Seeds
  Fresh, whole raw seeds and nuts: pecans, walnuts, cashews, and sunflowers.
  The use of peanuts and peanut butter is not encouraged, as these products often contain mold. If you do eat peanuts, get the type that is not hydrogenated—available in the baking supplies section of grocery store, not in the snack food or nut section.
- Eggs
- Grains, dried beans, rice
- Tofu
- Vegetables
  All fresh vegetables: carrots, broccoli, beans, etc. Cut carrots, celery, and peppers make nice snacks.
  Jicama (pronounced "hicama") is a root that is peeled and eaten as a crunchy snack ("Have some crunch with your lunch") or added to tossed salad. It is tasty and slightly sweet. Cut in strips and dip.
  Salads can be eaten with lemon, olive oil, and fresh garlic as dressing (instead of vinegar).
- Miscellaneous
  Salt, pepper, and herbs for seasoning—use caution because some herbs are old when purchased and can be moldy
  Tamari sauce

Recipes ·

Chicken Rice Soup

1 cup carrots, sliced
1-2 medium onions, chopped
3-4 stalks celery, sliced
1-3 garlic cloves, to taste
1 quart chicken broth
2 large chicken breasts cooked and chopped
1/2 cup uncooked brown rice
sea salt and pepper to taste

In large soup kettle, sauté the first four ingredients in olive oil. Add broth, chicken, brown rice, and two quarts water. Simmer on low heat until rice and vegetables are soft. Add sea salt and pepper to taste.

Hamburger Cabbage Soup

Brown in 8-quart stainless steel pot:
1 pound hamburger
1 large onion, diced
2 cups green beans, chopped
2 cups carrots, chopped
1 small turnip, diced
1-1/2 cups green pepper, chopped
1 large cabbage, chopped (cabbage has anti-cancer properties)
approximately 3 pints of water for liquid
minced garlic to taste
Spices: choose and add to taste 1/2 teaspoon of each: basil, thyme, dill weed, black pepper, and/or sea salt. Simmer all vegetables on low heat until tender.

Lentil Soup

1-1/2 cups washed lentils
Simmer in 3 cups water until tender
Combine and simmer until vegetables are tender:
2 cups green beans, chopped
1 cup green peppers, sliced
1 cup celery, chopped
1 cup parsnip (optional)
1 medium onion, diced
Spices: choose to your taste: sea salt, basil, black pepper, and/or thyme. Add water until desired thickness is reached.
    —Contributed by Terry Bateman

Basic Stir Fry

3 carrot sticks, sliced
1 cup string beans
1 cup cauliflower
1-2 cloves garlic
2 T. Canola oil
1 cup chicken broth thickened with 1 t. corn starch
salt and pepper to taste
Slightly brown garlic gloves in canola oil over medium heat. Add carrots, beans, and cauliflower and cook until tender. Lower heat and add chicken broth. Mix well and serve over boiled rice. Serves four.

Conclusion

In summary, CRC patients must modify their diets to include foods rich in vitamins and minerals. Knowledge of proper food combining, preparation, and an awareness of the possible contaminants in food will help the CRC patient in recovery.

Chapter Nine

Colon Cleansing Treatment and Candida Related Complex

An anti-CRC colon cleansing program was used in the study at the East West Clinic as one of the three foundation blocks for the treatment of Candida Related Complex (CRC). The other two foundation blocks were acupuncture (discussed in chapter Seven) and an anti-CRC diet (discussed in chapter Eight). The colon cleansing program consists of fungicides, intestinal cleansers, and friendly bacteria. This program expels CRC from the intestines, allowing the immune system to spring back and clean up CRC elsewhere in the body.

Fungicide's Role in Overcoming CRC

Although acupuncture is an important element in helping rid the body of CRC, it is limited in its ability to control the overgrowth of intestinal yeast. In a body infested with fungi, acupuncture can repair the systems and organs that are damaged. However, an equivalent of a pesticide (to kill the fungi) is also needed in order for the structure, or body, to stay intact. Hence, a fungicide is needed to directly kill the fungi infestation.

The safest and most effective fungicides seem to be those derived from natural botanical sources (i.e. caprylic acid/Caprol from coconut oil) rather than the chemical types developed in laboratories (for example, Nystatin). This may be because the CRC patient's immune system is so compromised that the body has difficulty assimilating any chemical, whether in food or in medications.

Colon in Relation to the Rest of the Body

It has often been stated that disease and death begin in the colon. A colon coated with a thick layer of built-up fecal material is a perfect breeding ground for fungi. It is this breeding ground which needs to be cleaned out so the Candida albicans are not able to live and multiply. Thus, one sees why a clean colon is essential in the battle against CRC. The average North American is carrying around from nine to twelve pounds of impacted fecal matter. A polluted colon produces toxins; the body then absorbs these toxins and poor health results. Additional fecal build-up means more toxins, and thus more illness.

Each portion of the colon has a direct relationship to the other body parts and functions. If there is pollution in part or all of the colon, illness results elsewhere in the body. Conversely, a clean colon means good health elsewhere in the body. In fact, various parts mirror the status of other parts of the body. For example, the condition of the colon and other body parts can be reflected in the eye's iris. And, likewise, the condition of the gallbladder and other body parts can be determined by examining the tongue. Basically, each part of the body is a microcosm of the whole body. Microcosm means a small part that is an epitome of the whole.

A book on one aspect of such mutual physical relationships, the face, is entitled *Your Face Never Lies* by Michio Kushi. It is written for the lay reader and makes fascinating reading. Kushi lists some additional examples of facial interrelatedness: the nose reflects the heart; the area above the upper lip reflects the sexual organs; the forehead reflects circulation, etc. [1] Thus, the face is similar to the colon in that it is also a microcosm of the whole body.

The ear can also be seen as a microcosm of the whole. As mentioned earlier in the acupuncture chapter, auricular medicine is based on the theory that there are 200 acupuncture points on the ear that relate to 200 parts of the body.

According to the *Alternative Health Guide*, the assumption behind iridology (the study of the iris) is that the condition of the iris of the eye gives indications which can be used in the diagnosis of mental and physical disorders throughout the body. The iris reflects other parts of the body as well. [2] Each pigment, fleck, and line have a special meaning to the iridologist. For more information on the topic of physical interrelatedness, refer to the *American Journal of Acupuncture*'s two-part series entitled "The Micro-Acupuncture System" from 1976, by Ralph Alan Dale, Ed.D., Ph.D. [3] In this series, Dr. Dale expands on this topic of how each part of the body is a microcosm of the whole.

Similarly, colon therapists believe that each section of the colon has a direct relationship to specific portions of the body. They believe that if there is fecal build-up in any section of the colon, a corresponding area of the body will suffer. See the chart on the next page.

For example, the cecum, the portion of the colon that forms the beginning of the large intestine, has a relationship to the pituitary gland. If the walls of the cecum are encrusted with fecal build-up, the pituitary gland will have a difficult time functioning. Pituitary gland disorders include: pituitary tumors, slow growth in children, hypoglycemia, and diabetes insipidus.

Another example: the midpoint of the transverse colon has a relationship to the lungs and bronchial tubes. If the walls of the transverse colon are encrusted or prolapsed (falling down out of position), then the lungs and bronchial tubes might experience difficulty (i.e. pneumonia and/or bronchial infections). Thus, colon therapists believe that cleansing the colon is "comparable to washing the skin; it has a profoundly positive effect on health." [4] So, not only is it desirable to cleanse the colon in order to remove toxic CRC-waste build-up, but it is also desirable for general good health.

A gentle, natural method of eliminating colon toxicity can be accomplished by using two natural agents: psyllium and bentonite. Neither one is absorbed into the system, but rather each adsorbs (it acts like a magnet) and then expels toxic materials in the feces. Both psyllium and bentonite are an integral part of the anti-CRC colon cleansing program used in the study at the East West Clinic.

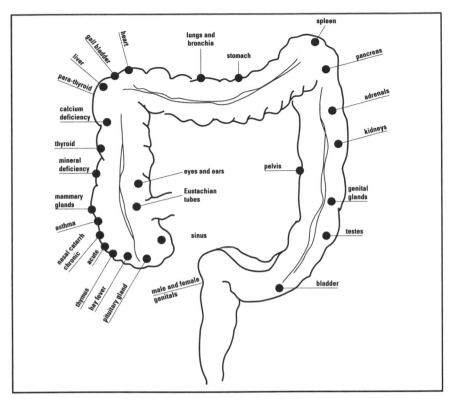

The normal colon with anatomical centers.

Over time, the accumulation of filth in the colon can be eradicated with the daily use of the psyllium/bentonite combination. Proper dietary modifications can help maintain a clean colon and reduce the likelihood of further toxic build-up.

Colon Therapy Ingredients

The ingredients used in the colon cleansing program consists of four items.

Anti-CRC Colon Cleansing Program
- Caprylic and oleic acids in olive oil, called Caprol
- Psyllium powder
- Liquid bentonite
- Beneficial bacteria

Caprylic acid is added to olive oil, which naturally has oleic acid in it. This mixture, called Caprol, is the portion of the program which is fungicidal, it kills the fungi on contact. Psyllium powder is an intestinal cleanser which works to clean the debris from the colon where the fungi breed. Bentonite is a detoxifier. It removes the toxic waste (CRC's poisonous by-product) from the body. And, finally, beneficial bacteria is reimplanted to replace those which have been lost, often due to antibiotics. These four items, mixed with just water (or half water and half unsweetened juice), make up the anti-CRC colon cleaning program.

Caprylic Acid and CRC

Caprol, containing liquid caprylic and oleic acids, is the fungicidal component of the anti-CRC colon cleansing program. Caprylic acid, a fatty acid, is a broad-spectrum anti-fungal agent effective against Candida albicans and other fungi, but harmless to friendly intestinal flora. It affects a direct assault upon the Candida albicans. It is a drugless approach which works independently of the host's defense mechanism.

Caprylic acid's anti-fungal properties were the subject of a study at the Japanese Niigata University School of Medicine: "the fungicidal effect of caprylic acid on Candida albicans was exceedingly powerful . . . Caprylic acid exhibits the most remarkable fungistatic and fungicidal properties of all normal saturated fatty acids with even-numbered carbon atoms studied." [5]

This information about caprylic acid's powerful antifungal properties was reported by the Japanese in 1961. However not until two decades later was it further discovered by a Canadian, Andrew Gutauskas, B.S. Pharmacy, that the benefits of caprylic acid are further enhanced when its transit through the intestinal tract is slowed. Caprylic acid must exert its fungicidal effect in the intestinal tract or not at all. The longer it can react, the better.

Unfortunately, caprylic acid is a substance that is normally quite rapidly absorbed into the intestinal tract and routed directly to the liver. There it is quickly metabolized and does not succeed at entering the general circulation. Just ten minutes after the oral intake of straight caprylic acid, more than 90% can be traced in the portal vein on its way to the liver. For this reason, the quite powerful caprylic acid has little anti-Candida albicans effect, both intestinally and systemically. This fact, however, is significantly altered if its absorption can be somehow slowed, allowing it to remain in the intestine for a longer period of time in order to complete its fungicidal mission. In this program, caprylic acid acquires its needed sustained-release properties from a gel, formed by the mixture of Caprol, colon cleansers, and water. This thick gel traps the caprylic acid and slows its transit through the colon.

Uncontrolled surges of caprylic acid into the liver are the most probable cause of adverse reactions to caprylic acid: however, while in this gelled state, caprylic acid does not escape into the liver. It is no surprise, then, that no adverse reactions to this gelled form of caprylic acid have been reported, even among individuals who previously reacted to other caprylic acid products.

Traditional caprylic acid preparations exist as capsules or tablets, but the preference is the liquid form. This mixing causes the caprylic acid to interact with the olive oil, thereby amplifying its fungicidal effects far beyond what caprylic acid has traditionally offered.

Oleic Acid and CRC

Oleic acid, the second acid ingredient in Caprol, is found naturally in olive oil. It, too, has significant CRC-battling effects. Normally harmless Candida albicans (if in small quantities) can convert, or mutate, into a disruptive mycelial form for several reasons — overuse of antibiotics being a prime example. When this happens, root-like tentacles are formed, which allow the new harmful fungi to penetrate the mucosa (or lining) of the intestinal wall and enter the bloodstream.

From there, the fungi easily gain access to other parts of the body. Oleic acid follows the mycelial, root-like tentacles of Candida albicans to the base of the root and kills it there. Oleic acid also hinders any additional conversion of Candida albicans yeast into its mycelial fungal form. Because of its invasive quality, the mycelial form of CRC must be eradicated if treatment is to be successful. As explained, oleic acid is of great importance in the destruction of CRC.

Olive Oil Benefits

Caprol (olive oil with added caprylic acid) was designed to take advantage of the additional health benefits of olive oil. A study of almost 5,000 Italians in the *Journal of the American Medical Association* discovered that olive oil, especially when used on prepared foods in place of butter, is linked to lower blood pressure, blood sugar, and cholesterol levels. [6] So, not only does Caprol have antifungal properties, it is also linked to lower blood pressure, blood sugar, and cholesterol levels due to its olive oil component.

The rate of release of caprylic acid is independent of the patient's intestinal pH condition. The gel, by trapping the caprylic acid, unilaterally establishes the proper gelled conditions for a suitable rate of release of caprylic acid.

In the study at the East West Clinic, Garlic, OxyCleanse and grapefruit seed extract were used alternately with Caprol when symptoms persisted beyond two to three months. This was done to insure that fungi that mutated and became resistant to one form could be controlled.

Psyllium and CRC

Psyllium (pronounced "silly-um") is the second part of the anti-CRC colon cleansing program and a key element in deriving the needed gelled consistency which slowly moves caprylic acid through the intestinal tract. There are two parts of the psyllium that are useful in cleansing the colon: the seeds and the husks. The seeds, even when crushed into a powder, still retain tiny granules, which scrape away the accumulated fecal build-up on the colon wall. The husks absorb water and form the gel, retarding the passage of the fungicidal caprylic acid.

Psyllium is a plant grown commercially in India and its husk is used as a bulk-forming laxative in numerous products. These husks expand when mixed with liquid, creating a roughage-like gelled substance. The expanding bulk cleans out the pockets lining the colon wall. It is estimated that 80% of the North American population over 40 years old have diverticulosis, a ballooning of tiny sacs or pockets on the intestinal wall. These tiny pockets collect fecal matter, which further accelerates pollution of the colon and these diverticula provide a ripe breeding ground for Candida albicans.

Constance Kies, Ph.D., states, "As it (psyllium) absorbs water in the digestive tract, the psyllium expands, stimulating and speeding up elimination." [7] Psyllium is also a cholesterol fighter, as Kies found in an experiment with healthy volunteers. The cholesterol levels of the subjects studied dropped, on average, from 193 to 168 when they added psyllium to their customary diets.

The intake of psyllium also reduces toxic overload. This reaction occurs when poisons are released by dead and dying fungi (referred to as the "die-off reaction") associated with the eradication of CRC. The toxic overload is a result of the successful killing of the Candida albicans fungus by the fungicidal Caprol. The psyllium gel absorbs these toxins from the colon and carries them out of the system.

In fact, gastroenterologist Jack D. Welch, M.D., at the University of Oklahoma Health Sciences Center, notes in his research that psyllium entirely prevents the expected fungal "die-off" reaction of gas pain and nausea. [8] When a large number of Candida albicans are killed off during the initial period of treatment, a great amount of toxic material is suddenly released. As these toxins lie in the gastrointestinal tract, they can cause flu-like symptoms.

The psyllium seed fragments are very hard; they tend to scrape away at the toxic deposits on the walls of the intestines. If the scraping psyllium seed powder is added to the bulk-forming power of the psyllium husk powder in the proper ratio, the preparation becomes an intestinal cleanser, sweeping the dead fungi down to the lower bowels where they are finally eliminated. This cleansing process may take a period of months, depending on several factors such as the severity and length of the CRC, the strength of the immune system, and how well the patient avoids the initial cause of CRC.

One can now easily see why a psyllium product containing both seeds and husks is preferred. Most psyllium products are husks only and sold solely for their laxative effect. This husks-only psyllium possesses minimal intestinal cleansing action, because it lacks powdered psyllium seeds.

The anti-CRC colon cleansing program suggested in this book uses the dual benefits of both psyllium seeds and husks. The addition of seeds is a complicated process. Psyllium seeds are very hard and difficult to grind into a powder. This adds further costs, due to labor and machinery expenses associated with grinding the seeds and mixing them in with the powdered husks.

Psyllium has a much greater concentration of healthy fiber than oat bran. This high fiber content can significantly reduce harmfully high levels of cholesterol. Oat bran is about 14% fiber, half of which is soluble (capable of dissolving in water), while psyllium is 96% fiber, 85% of which is soluble. A short-term (just 20 weeks) University of Minnesota study found that only one teaspoon of powdered psyllium husks, taken three times a day, lowered cholesterol by about 6%—a significant drop. [9]

Dr. James Anderson, a medical and clinical nutrition professor at the University of Kentucky, "supports the idea of making psyllium more widely available in food products to give consumers a variety of choices for lowering their cholesterol through dietary measures." [10] Thus, researchers have seen the benefits of psyllium and are urging its wider use.

Bentonite and CRC

Bentonite is the third part of the colon cleansing program developed to eliminate CRC from the body. Bentonite, a volcanic ash found in the Black Hills of South Dakota, is an inert mineral silicate. When processed into a very fine powder and suspended in distilled water, bentonite adsorbs (acts like a magnet pulling toxins to it) intestinal waste products without being absorbed into the system. It just passes through the intestinal tract attaching the toxins to itself. This action is similar to fly paper and flies.

The unique properties of bentonite were reported by Frederic Damrau, M.D., who established that bentonite adsorbs toxins both in laboratory dishes and in humans. Because bentonite itself is not absorbed into the body, whatever it adsorbs is removed in the feces. [11] Bentonite provides an excellent vehicle for removing miscellaneous intestinal poisons and toxins generated by Candida albicans.

Bentonite must be in a liquid form in order to exert optimal effect. If taken in powder or tablet form, the digestive system must then convert it to liquid form. This task is not likely, however, because bentonite does not mix easily with water. Furthermore, the digestive system does not have the equipment to accomplish this function. Therefore ingestion of bentonite in liquid form is strongly recommended.

Beneficial Bacteria and CRC

Reimplanting beneficial bacteria is the fourth part of the colon cleansing program for ridding CRC from the body. Beneficial bacteria needs to be reimplanted in the colon to help provide equilibrium in the intestinal tract — a balance between friendly and harmful bacteria. This balance was lost when the fungi proliferated. New beneficial bacteria will also aid in arresting further intestinal CRC.

Beneficial bacteria are needed for the digestion of foods. There are different types of this beneficial bacteria used in the anti-CRC colon cleansing program, including acidophilus, bifidus, laterosporus, and S. faucium. These bacteria produce acidophilin (a natural antibiotic), lactic acid (which aids lactose digestion), and hydrogen peroxide (which adds life-giving oxygen). Beneficial bacteria is effective against disease-causing bacteria. This reimplantation strengthens the immune system by lessening its workload.

A billion or more cells of beneficial bacteria are included in each capsule. This seems excessive, however it is necessary to ingest many cells because "it takes approximately one million therapeutic-strength acidophilus (cells) to control a single yeast cell . . ." as reported by Dalton Moore, C.H., a Canadian Candida consultant. [12]

The presence of food in the stomach activates stomach acids, which kill the beneficial bacteria. So the colon cleansing program must be ingested on an empty stomach to preserve the beneficial bacteria. The term "pH" is the symbol expressing the degree of alkalinity or acidity. "These acids (when food is being digested) could be a pH level of 1.0 to 2.0. Friendly bacteria work best in an environment with a pH of approximately 4.5 to 5.5, which are normal pH levels found in a healthy colon." [13] "Taking it (beneficial bacteria) on an empty stomach will minimize loss (of good bacteria) due to the stomach acids present when food is being digested," states Moore. [14]

An added benefit of ingesting beneficial bacteria is a lessening of food allergies. A British doctor, J. O. Hunter, hypothesizes that patients with food intolerance (allergies) have an abnormal gut flora. [15] Restoring this bacterial balance to its proper levels can greatly improve a CRC patient's tolerance for food.

Water and the Anti-CRC Colon Cleansing Program

When mixing this anti-CRC colon cleansing program, it is recommended that purified, distilled water be used. Common tap water contains chlorine which will completely negate the benefit of the beneficial bacteria in the colon cleansing program. "Chlorine kills bacteria in swimming pools and will do the same to your friendly flora," says Moore. [16]

Cleansing Action in the Intestinal Tract

Once the mixture is ingested, it causes unique and beneficial occurrences to take place in the CRC-diseased digestive tract. First, the liquid caprylic acid is released into the intestinal wall at a slowed rate. This is due to the gelled nature of the psyllium component, not to the intestinal pH conditions of acidity or alkalinity, which vary widely among individuals. Consequently, results are predictable, consistent, and favorable. Caprylic acid is slowly released through the entire length of the fungi-infested intestinal tract at a predictable rate controlled by the gel.

Next, as the gel rubs itself against the intestinal wall, it acts as a paint brush covering the wall with the liquid caprylic acid. Not a square millimeter of wall is missed throughout the entire length of the intestines.

Because the Candida albicans microorganisms are buried deep within the toxic accumulations on the intestinal walls, access to them is difficult. But the bulking action of the gel forcibly rubs liquid caprylic acid into the filth and onto the Candida albicans, thus effectively reaching and killing the fungi.

The liquid bentonite adsorbs the imbedded fungi and removes them from the system. A healthy beneficial bacteria is restored through implantation of new cells.

Recipe and Mixing Instructions

Anti-CRC Colon Cleansing Program

The four-part colon cleansing program used in the study at the East West Clinic included the four previously described ingredients of Caprol, psyllium, bentonite, and beneficial bacteria (acidophilus) dispersed in water.

Caprol consists of olive oil (including oleic acid) with added liquid caprylic acid, a natural product derived from coconut oil which has strong fungicidal properties.

Psyllium powder is made from high-grade psyllium seeds and husks. This powdered product provides expansive, adhesive bulk. Bulk is important to the colonic system because it helps move the material through the colon. Using a psyllium with both powdered seeds and husks helps clean out the fecal buildup in the cracks and crevices of the colon wall.

Bentonite is an adsorbent detoxifying product that is considered beneficial to the natural functioning of the intestinal wall by drawing (like a magnet) toxins to it and flushing them out of the system.

Beneficial bacteria reimplants decimated friendly flora into the colon, helping to maintain a proper equilibrium balance between friendly and harmful bacteria in the intestinal tract.

Suggested usage is twice daily. Take one-half hour before breakfast, and again two hours after (or one hour before) supper. It is important to take this mixture on an empty stomach. If taken when there is food in the stomach, the acids stimulated by the food will kill the beneficial bacteria and negate that part of the program.

Mixing Instructions

Using a two to four cup jar with a tight fitting lid, add the above ingredients in the order listed below. By adding ingredients in this order, items will mix together more easily without lumping. Drink immediately. If even a short delay occurs, mixture will thicken, making drinking difficult. The mixture is designed to thicken and expand in the intestinal tract. It will thicken and expand in the jar even if not ingested, so drink quickly.

Ingredients

Water:	8 ounces, or 1 cup, at room temperature. Distilled preferred. (Half and half unsweetened juice and water may be used if water alone is not tolerated well.)
Bentonite:	1 to 2 tablespoons. Shake bottle before pouring.
Caprol:	1/2 teaspoon to 1 tablespoon (see below)
Beneficial Bacteria: (example: Acidophilus)	Contents of 1 to 2 capsules. Lightly massage the capsule between the fingers prior to opening, so that it can be easily pulled apart.
Psyllium:	1 heaping teaspoon. Add last.

Screw on the jar lid and shake vigorously for 10 to 15 seconds. Drink immediately, as mixture thickens very quickly.

Severely Infected-CRC Patients

Week 1: Start with just psyllium and bentonite.
Week 2: Add 1/2 teaspoon Caprol to psyllium/bentonite combination.
Week 3: Increase Caprol to 1 teaspoon.
Week 4: Increase Caprol to 2 teaspoons.
Week 5: Increase Caprol to 3 teaspoons (equal to one tablespoon)

Caprol is a fungicide. If die-off reaction (nausea and/or flu-like symptoms) is severe when beginning the program, cut back on this portion of the program. After a week, begin reintroducing it gradually, increasing 1/2 teaspoon per week until up to 1 tablespoon.

The patient should feel free to experiment with usage to fit individual physiological reactions.

Psyllium has a stool loosening effect while bentonite has a stool tightening effect. Thus, if the patient tends to have loose stools, 2 tablespoons of bentonite are recommended. If, on the other hand, the patient tends toward constipation, less bentonite and more psyllium is recommended.

The mixture has a bland taste. Some people drink as above. Others have found that adding granulated wheat or barley green enhances this program. Still others substitute unsweetened fruit juice for all or part of the water.

Finishing the Colon Cleansing Program

For many CRC patients, the wellness experienced from using the program will not last unless they continue with the psyllium (intestinal cleanser) and bentonite (intestinal detoxicant) combination for at least another ten months. Adding Caprol to the psyllium/bentonite mixture every third week, for a period of five days is also recommended. Following the anti-CRC diet will also aid in achieving improved health.

If, however, the person is subjected to antibiotics, excesses of the wrong kinds of foods, or extreme stress, its very probable that there could be a recurrence of the Candida albicans overgrowth. The patient may need to return to the program temporarily. Whether the patient will have to return to the program depends on how well the patient is able to avoid what initially caused the systemic overgrowth of the Candida albicans.

Die-Off Reaction

Many patients with CRC, but not all, experience uncomfortable effects within the first week, often commencing on the second day following the beginning of treatment. These effects may include flu-like symptoms (stuffiness, headache, general achiness, or diarrhea), skin rashes, heavy limbs, vaginal irritation and/or discharge, unusual numbness in the legs, or possibly even mental confusion. The exact die-off symptoms are many and varied. These symptoms result from the release of toxins from rapidly dying Candida albicans in the colon. The exact symptoms depend upon the individual case and are sometimes dramatic. The die-off reaction normally lasts from one day to no longer than one week.

It may be necessary to cut back dosages of the fungicidal components of the program, the Caprol and beneficial bacteria (which also attack the harmful fungi), until symptoms subside. When die-off symptoms subside, increase these two components gradually over a few weeks to the recommended level.

One of the best features of this program is that the normal die-off reaction, if any, is relieved to a very great extent by the detoxifying action of both the psyllium and bentonite components. Taking extra vitamin C and E also help alleviate the symptoms.

Benefits of the CRC Cleansing Program

Besides cleaning the colon, eradicating CRC, and improving health, there are additional benefits to the colon cleansing program. Author Dennis Hunt, M.D., in his book *No More Cravings*, has successfully treated CRC and says "some patients are having fewer weight problems, less water retention, and an absence of cravings . . ." [17] Dr. Hunt feels that this aspect of CRC should be of prime importance to bariatricians (specialists in weight control).

Conclusion

In summary, the four-part anti-CRC colon cleansing program is effective in treating patients with both short-term and long-term CRC. Acupuncture is an important element of healing, but an anti-fungal program is needed as well. This program consists of Caprol, psyllium, bentonite, and beneficial bacteria. A thorough colon cleansing will rid the body of toxic waste and promote good health elsewhere in the body.

Case Study Five

43-Year-Old Male: Back from the Brink of Suicide

In October of 1983, I was helping a friend roof his house. While lifting heavy bundles of shingles, I noticed discomfort in my groin and urinary tract for the first time in my life. This discomfort was transient and passed with rest. So I ignored it and kept on with my life as usual, working as a chiropractor in my Missouri office. I was about 30 pounds overweight, a heavy drinker, ate lots of hamburgers, potato chips, cookies, and drank glass after glass of iced tea.

By January of 1984, the problem with my urinary tract that had previously come and gone had now come to stay! I literally had pain and discomfort every waking hour. For some reason, thank God, I could sleep at night with no trouble, but during the day I experienced agonizing, constant pain—especially with any activity.

By March of 1984, the problem had not gone away so I decided to consult a specialist. He said, "Nothing is wrong. You'll just have to ride it out." Mentally, I felt better knowing it wasn't cancer or a tumor, but I STILL HURT!

In April of that same year, my wife and I took a vacation in Florida, but I hurt so bad the whole week I couldn't enjoy our vacation at all. On Friday of that vacation week, I finally gave up and consulted a skin doctor, who put me on prednisone. I had two days of blessed relief and then it was bad again. I decided to be patient and just ride it out.

When I was still not better by November, seven months later, I decided to spend $1,000 in an attempt to find the source of the pain. A urologist put me in the hospital for a day to perform a uroscopy and dilation. He said he couldn't find anything and that I should get back in touch with him if I was not better after the dilation. Seeing no improvement, I realized I had spent $1,000 for nothing.

In January and February of 1985, I consulted a couple of chiropractors. One was Dr. Chuck Anderson, D.C., who ordered some blood tests. He then said I had Candida albicans. I didn't know it at that time, but his diagnosis was correct. However, his recommended treatment was not helpful. It consisted of a few vitamins, exercise, and radical diet changes. He was on the right track, but I guess his treatment was lacking. I went back to my Merck's Manual, and sure enough it painted the exact picture of my signs and symptoms under the category of

Candida albicans. From that time on, I was convinced I had a fungus infection. But, oh my, what an incredible challenge to cut out all junk food, sugar, and yeast!! I only lasted a short five weeks on the strict diet. I did continue with my exercise, running several miles every morning (pain or no pain) but I still showed no improvement.

I had a patient/friend whom I called "Mr. Ed." We were chatting one day and I shared my problem with him. He said, "Doc, I'll treat you with reflexology and massage!" I said, "O.K., I have nothing to lose." So, he treated me two or three times a week. His treatments never did much, but he sure did encourage me. This kept me going. He really seemed to care about what happened to me and worked hard on me, often performing hour-long treatments.

By November of 1985, I decided again that it was time to consult a doctor. So I went to a neurologist. He ran $1,000 worth of tests on me and said I was perfectly normal! Of course, I knew better. I was beginning to get very depressed, feeling helpless and discouraged. But I kept up the search.

In December of 1985 and on into January of 1986, I began running cultures of my urinary tract. I found a great deal of streptococci and staphylococci. I then started a round of antibiotics. I was elated when I got well, but that only lasted for a little more than a week. After that I was worse than ever. So, in February, I went to the hospital in town and a medical doctor there put me on intravenous antibiotics. This cost me $2,000 and it was all for naught! It didn't do anything to help my problem. By April, I headed for the Columbia Regional Hospital. I consulted with a neurosurgeon who said he could cut the nerves to the groin and urinary tract but he didn't want to. Thank the Lord for his reluctance. Another doctor I saw, a skin specialist, also could not help me.

In May, I consulted a surgeon in town who said I was depressed. He put me on antidepressants, which did not help my situation. But, I began hoarding the pills. I thought if I didn't get relief soon, I was going to end it all! I was literally suicidal.

In June, a proctologist ordered an X-ray. After reading it, he said I was normal. In October, after performing blood work, an osteopath told me I had allergies. Her treatment, like the others, again did nothing.

In December, I traveled 170 miles to Barnes Hospital in St. Louis—a massive place with many doctors. After hours of waiting, I finally got to see a doctor. He put me on Bactrim. From that, I got one day of relief, but that was all.

All this time I continued exercising and running. In February of 1987, I joined the gym in town and continued to work out hard—weights, bicycle, and running. I had to get rid of this problem and I knew exercise was good for me. So, hurting or not, I kept it up.

By April of 1987, I had to do something. So, off to the Mayo Clinic I went. After a week there (at a cost of $1,300), they said I needed a psychiatrist! I was frustrated with the expense, the lack of answers, and, most of all, the unrelenting pain. It was all so incredible. I compromised and went to a psychologist. He told me I definitely had a physical problem, but now it was affecting me in my psyche. He referred me to a pain control clinic in Springfield, 240 miles to the south of my home. I spent two weeks there and spent $5,000; again for nothing. It was awful.

The pain continued. I began to listen hour after hour to subliminal tapes. I finally realized that they did nothing to help me. I then tried subliminal videos but they made me worse.

By August, I decided to try another approach. I heard that a clinic in Excelsior Springs gave prostate injections. It would be very painful, but they assured me that they would probably help me. I took the injections, but I got worse! I drove close to 300 miles, round trip, three times a week for almost a month for more of nothing.

By November of 1987, I began to turn to God. I decided to fast and pray. After seventeen days without any food (I had chosen to skip the prayer part), I was 20 pounds lighter, very weak (could barely walk), and yet with continuous pain. I was mortified, but I still didn't give up.

By March of 1988, I thought I would go to the Gonstead Chiropractic Clinic in Wisconsin. Maybe, I thought, I had something wrong with my spine and tailbone. After a week at the clinic, there was no change.

So, when I returned home, I began reading Dr. Norman Walker's books on colon health. I decided then to change my eating habits radically and to take some colonics. These did help some. So, I believed I was on the right tract. After a weekly colonic for three months and no junk food, I felt some better from time to time. Some afternoons I would have mild relief, but at night the pain would be worse again. This cycle of mild relief followed by more pain continued. It was still awfully discouraging and frustrating. But I hung in there.

By August of 1988, I had consulted another osteopath who recommended DMSO injections into the bladder. After about seven injections, I realized they were a waste of time.

Two months later, I returned to the proctologist who said I should have an ultrasound on my prostate and a biopsy. It cost another $1,000 to find out I had benign prostatic hypertrophy (a non-cancerous increase in the size of the prostrate gland)—BIG DEAL!

By now I had tried so many doctors and medications, I had lost count. Besides the antibiotics, both oral and intravenous, including Flagyl and anti-fungal drugs including Nyzoral, Nystatin, and Ketacozanole. The antibiotics helped for a few days then the symptoms returned worse than ever, but the other drugs produced no change in my symptoms. I was suffering with the symptoms related to the continuous bladder infection, including fatigue, anxiety, irritability, food sensitivities, abdominal bloating, and poor concentration.

In December of 1988, I found a church I liked with people who really believed that God answers prayer. During a service, I went forward for prayer. This, I truly believe, was the turning point. As we prayed, we believed, I mean we really believed! Something had to be done and soon.

By now, I had spent in excess of $15,000 on treatments for my problem, which were all a total waste of time and money. None of this money was reimbursed by insurance. This money all came out of my own pocket.

We continued to pray on into the spring of 1989. By July, I decided to really get serious and this time pray as well as fast. I went 28 days without food, just drinking fresh juices, and added lots of prayer. I had confidence God would tell me the answer to my problem. At the end of the fast, I saw an ad in a *National*

Health Freedom magazine for an anti-Candida program consisting of Caprol with caprylic acid, psyllium, bentonite, and acidophilus. This was now August of 1989, totaling almost six long years of suffering excruciating pain every waking hour in my urinary tract. I thought to myself, "this looks like it's at least worth a try. What the heck, I'll order it."

I started on the program August 7, 1989. I'll never forget that moment. Within a few days, I began to notice a little relief, so I was hopeful. Within a week, improvement started, albeit slight. In my own mind, I believe that I had finally found the answer to my prayers. There was a significant lessening of pain and inflammation. My bowel elimination improved in function significantly.

After a few months, I had a noticeable relief; not anywhere near complete, but better than I had been in a long time. With the anti-Candida program, diet changes, and walking, I lost the desired 25 pounds. I knew then that I was on the right track. It was a godsend.

I was encouraged but I also needed to be careful about my diet. I knew I couldn't go back to the sugar, yeast, or junk food without trouble, so I had to continue to adhere very strictly to the diet and exercise. I had lots of fresh fruits, vegetables, whole grains, lean meat, water, diet Coke (it never bothered me), and plenty of daily exercise. It was hard, but was I happy. I was on the road to recovery. I took a daily double dose of the anti-Candida program between August of 1989 and March 1991. After one and three quarters of a year, I felt sufficiently improved to be able to cut down to one dose a day. I continued on that daily single dose religiously until April of 1993 when I quit altogether. I had been on the program for three years and eight months.

Today I am almost 100% well, with only occasional, minimal discomfort. My diet consists of an abundance of fresh, raw fruits, some vegetables, occasional lean meat, and whole grains. I drink mineral water, some diet Coke, very weak coffee, and, once in a while, some fresh fruit juice. But I never have any sugar, white flour, yeast (bread with yeast), or corn syrup. I also stay away from condiments with sugar and vinegar. I don't indulge in alcohol or smoking and don't use any prescription drugs.

I can only say that a Candida infection is a living hell that I wouldn't wish on my worst enemy. Let me tell you, I took my health for granted for 33 years but I don't anymore. So, whether I live to be 45 (I'm 43 now) or 100, I'm going to be as healthy as I can be. Lots of people say, "well, I have to die of something." To die is one thing. To suffer for the last 40 years of your life is quite another. What good is it to live to a certain age if you are sick and miserable half the time? People put so much emphasis on figuring out disease, but I say 95% of the time in the U.S.A., you can forget the disease. Concentrate on what you must do to be healthy. I suggest exercise, strict eating habits (preferably uncooked food), regular chiropractic adjustments, ample prayer, and good thoughts—trusting in the Lord and not worrying. Keep your weight down and get enough rest. Keep the colon immaculately clean and get plenty of sunshine and fresh air. Follow these suggestions and you won't get sick. It's really very simple if only people would just do it.

Well, that's my story. I hope it will help someone. It if helps just one person, it will be worth the trouble of writing it down.

In the Name of Jesus,
—Dr. Kevin B. Keough, Riobamba, Ecuador

P.S. Now instead of ending up committing suicide or some other crazy thing, we are serving the Lord full-time on the mission field in Ecuador—in perfect health. I am excited about how He has turned my life around! And, God bless you, Colet, for caring enough to try to reach people with this treatment. I wish I could tell you how prevalent this problem is in Ecuador, but I don't really know. In the past eight months, we've seen a few cases, but not many. I just really can't say with certainty, and I doubt if anyone else here cares. Most problems here are worms and parasites.

Chapter Ten

Other Natural Therapies That Also Help CRC Recovery

There are other natural therapies — in addition to the anti-CRC colon cleansing program mentioned in chapter nine — that help in waging the war against Candida Related Complex (CRC). These include herbs, vitamins, minerals, essential oils, colonics, exercise, and specific foods, such as garlic.

Alternative health care professionals have been successfully using natural therapies to keep harmful bacteria and fungi in check for years, thus avoiding antibiotics and their resultant immune-suppressing effects.

"Most doctors no longer use Nystatin (a prescription antifungal drug) or antibiotics," writes James Balch, M.D., and Phyllis Balch, C.N.C., authors of the book entitled *Prescription for Nutritional Healing*. [1] They believe the discontinuance or, at least the reduction, in prescribing Nystatin and antibiotics is "because they weaken the immune system and can damage certain organs . . . Stronger strains of yeast can develop, becoming resistant to the drugs. Higher doses are then required, further weakening the immune system." The use of prescription anti-fungal drugs to fight CRC often produces only a short-term respite. In fact, some doctors have turned from drugs to natural therapies in order to treat CRC, but unfortunately many still favor drug intervention.

Science reported on CRC, stating that fungi are becoming resistant to the azoles (i.e. ketoconazoles, fluconazoles, and itraconazoles): "The overall effect is fungistatic rather than fungicidal, limiting the utility of these drugs." [2] This means that fungi merely become inactive, rather than being killed.

In addition to feeling that natural therapies should be used to fight CRC (because of their long-term success in this area), the Balchs also agree that various natural therapies need to be rotated due to fungal resistance, although not as rapidly as drugs. Thus, rotating natural treatment programs is beneficial. [3] It is helpful to have various types of ammunition in the arsenal against CRC.

Other health care professionals feel that not only should natural therapies be rotated, but the question of why the body succumbs to CRC in the first place should be researched. Nutritionist Larry Wilson, M.D., writes that it is "a common practice and mistake to treat yeast symptomatically as a 'disease,' without paying attention to underlying biochemical weaknesses that are causing suscepti-bility to yeast infection." [4] He identifies four contributing factors to CRC:

1. Copper imbalance, either a deficiency or an excess
2. Sodium potassium ratio less than 2.5:1, showing degree of stress
3. Sugar and carbohydrate intolerance
4. Over-alkaline body chemistry, with resultant digestion problems

If the underlying biochemical weaknesses are discovered, they can be correct-ed. This will aid in the struggle against CRC and the prevention of a recurrence.

Although the study at the East West Clinic did not use all the following natur-al therapies on a routine basis, natural therapies were used alternately with the anti-CRC colon cleansing program mentioned in chapter nine.

Herbs

Herbal therapy, used for centuries in Eastern cultures, is effective in treating fungal infections, as well as a host of other complaints. Herbal therapy accom-plishes this while avoiding rapid drug resistance and toxic reactions, which are often side effects of antifungal pharmaceutical medications.

Candida albicans can quickly and readily become drug resistant, so it is imperative to explore alternative therapies. "Single agent chemotherapy (treat-ment of infections or tumors with chemicals as opposed to natural therapy) may be effective for a short period of time, but generally the fungi become resistant to the medications rather quickly," states M. M. Van Benschoten, O.M.D. [5] He continues: "Herbal therapy has a much greater potential for producing long-term amelioration (improvement) of systemic fungal infections, as the complex chemi-cal nature of botanical substances (herbs), and the simultaneous use of several different antifungal herbs makes the development of resistance more unlikely." [6] Natural anti-fungal therapies are more effective than drugs because botanical substances or natural herbs have a more complex chemical nature than do sin-gle-agent pharmaceuticals. This makes it more difficult for the fungi to mutate and become resistant to the complexity of natural therapies.

There are hundreds of herbs used for their therapeutic value. Michael A. Weiner, Ph.D., in his book *The People's Herbal: A Family Guide to Herbal Home Remedies*, writes about symptoms and illnesses, and herbs and herbal recipes that assist in recovery.

Dr. Weiner is educated in nutritional ethno-medicine and his book identifies various herbs that alter the process of nutrition and excretion, expel intestinal worms, prevent the formation of gall and kidney stones, relieve rheumatism, fight infection, expel gas, evacuate bowels, clean the blood, increase urine out-put, reduce fever, calm nerves, encourage wound healing, and induce vomiting. [7]

In fact, many people are already using herbal medicine without even realizing it. For example, most homes have a bottle of Ipecac, an herbal preparation, in the medicine chest in case of accidental poisoning. Many of the above symptoms mentioned by Dr. Weiner are experienced by CRC patients and these patients would probably find that studying this book would be helpful.

Dr. Van Benschoten feels, when using herbal remedies in dealing with CRC, that there are four points that should be addressed. Different herbal remedies correct specific CRC-weakened areas. They are as follows:

1. Removing damp/heat (swelling and inflammation)
   Remedy: gentian combination, Coptis, and scute combination;
2. Regulating Qi (chi) (abdominal distension, constipation, and bloating)
   Remedy: linum and rhubarb combination, areca seed combination;
3. Tonifying Qi (weakness, poor appetite, and indigestion)
   Remedy: pinellia and ginseng six combination;
4. Warming interior (abdominal pain relieved by heat)
   Remedy: cardamom and fennel combination. [8]

Although there can be a multiplicity of symptoms in the CRC patient, there are several most common complaints. Dr. Van Benschoten believes that various body organs/functions can be specifically targeted in order to maximize CRC therapy: for problems in genital organs, use dictamnus, gentiana, and philodendron; for the digestive tract, use Qi (chi) regulators and tonifiers; for liver problems, use citrus reticulate, paeonia alba, and gardenia, and if the nervous system has problems, use xanthium, angelica dahurica, and Mentha. [9] The CRC patient, when overwhelmed with their own ailments, can take comfort in the knowledge that various herbs can help them.

Herbal Teas

The use of herbal teas in conjunction with acupuncture therapy produces certain predictable outcomes. For example, as noted above, there are herbal teas that remove dampness (reduce swelling from fluid retention), strengthen chi, drain chi, and warm individuals with cold patterns.

One special herbal tea is advocated by many health care professionals for treatment of CRC. Pau d'arco, the inner bark of the taheebo tree, aids the CRC patient by helping resist the spread of Candida albicans through the blood. [10] It is also an antibacterial agent, has a healing effect, and cleanses the blood. [11]

Vitamins

A medical dictionary defines vitamins as "organic compounds or chemicals, found in various foodstuff, necessary for the maintenance of normal life." [12] Surprising as this may be, the word "vitamin" was only invented in 1911. [13] Vitamins were lettered alphabetically in the order in which they are discovered.

The Balchs describe vitamins as contributing "to good health by regulating the metabolism and assisting the biochemical processes that release energy from digested food." [14] Most CRC patients have a vitamin deficiency, because the fecal build-up on the intestinal wall prevents nutrients from being absorbed. This creates a chronic nutritional deficiency which causes many of the CRC symptoms. Symptoms that can be exhibited by the vitamin-deficient person are listed below.

Vitamin-Deficiency Symptoms

Vitamin A: retards growth in children, impairs vision, and increases susceptibility to infection

Vitamin B1: numbness, tingling, burning in feet and leg muscles, can escalate into leg swelling, heart enlargement, and circulatory collapse

Vitamin B2: cracking of skin at mouth corners, chapped hands, dry scaly skin, and irritation of eyes

Vitamin B3:	dermatitis, diarrhea, and dementia
Vitamin B6:	infants only, convulsions, stunted growth, and anemia
Vitamin B12:	severe anemia and nervous system disorders
Vitamin C:	scurvy, irritability, bleeding from gums, anemia, and heart problems.
Vitamin D:	bone abnormalities in children
Vitamin E:	premature aging, anemia, and difficulty walking
Vitamin K:	hemorrhages [15, 16]

If a symptom exists, supplementation can help to correct the CRC-induced deficiency.

Almost fifty years ago, the U.S. Food and Nutrition Board established the Recommended Dietary Allowance (RDA) for vitamin intake. [17] Then, in 1974, the U.S. Food and Drug Administration established the Recommended Daily Allowance for vitamin intake which is used for product labeling. [18] Unfortunately, the amounts these governmental agencies decided upon only defines the bare minimum to ward off disease. The RDA does not take into account the amounts of vitamins needed to provide optimal health. Alternative health therapists believe an Optimum Daily Allowance (ODA) of larger doses of vitamins should be recommended for maximum health. For example, the RDA for Vitamin A is 5,000 international units (IU) and the ODA for this same vitamin is from 10,000 to 50,000 IU. [19, 20]

According to nutritionist Larry Wilson, M.D., author of *Nutritional Balancing and Hair Mineral Analysis*, sufficient vitamin intake is an important element missing in most of our diets. He believes vitamins can be used, not only to cure certain diseases, but to also help the body remove toxic metals and increase energy:

> A serious misconception is the belief that vitamins are only useful for eliminating deficiency diseases. A second mistake is the idea that one can obtain adequate vitamin nutrition from the average American diet. Today many people have numerous subclinical deficiencies and vague complaints that clear up when extra vitamins are taken. Vitamins can also be used as therapeutic agents to alter body chemistry, remove toxic metals, and enhance energy production. [21]

This aspect of natural therapy is too important to ignore, especially for the CRC patient.

Minerals

The body needs minerals for sustaining bones and blood, maintaining a proper composition of fluids, and maintaining a healthy nervous system. Minerals are divided into two types: bulk and trace. Bulk minerals include calcium, magnesium, phosphorus, potassium, sodium and sulfur. Trace minerals include copper, fluoride, iodine, iron, manganese, selenium, and zinc. [22]

Often the CRC patient will exhibit certain mineral deficiencies. For example, a copper deficiency will encourage CRC. Copper is a natural fungus fighter used to spray fruits and vegetables. It is also added to swimming pools to retard the spread of fungi. Many prescribed medications adversely affect the body's proper physiological copper balance. Birth control pills, steroid drugs, and antibiotics are three such drugs which deplete the body of copper and allow the yeast to grow unchecked. [23] Dr. Wilson's book clearly links a copper deficiency to the severe consequences of a CRC-ridden individual.

As mentioned earlier, a deficiency in chromium is also often associated with CRC patients. Chromium is an energizer and a blood stabilizer. It is believed that this mineral helps transport and attach insulin to the cell walls. An individual who has a chromium deficiency will crave sugar, experience fatigue, and have mood swings.

CRC patients can greatly improve their health by achieving and maintaining proper mineral levels in their bodies.

Essential Oils

Essential oils are the essence, in liquid form, of plants, shrubs, flowers, trees, roots, bushes, and seeds. For pure, effective essential oils, a great deal of the original source must be used to generate a very small amount of oil. For instance, 6,000 pounds of the Melissa plant produce one pound of melissa oil, and 5,000 pounds of rose petals produce only one pound of rose oil. This means that the oils are very expensive. However, only a few drops are needed for a therapeutic effect. It is important to note that if essential oils are diluted to reduce the expense, then they are not as effective.

Studies of essential oils show that these oils may help create an environment in which fungus, harmful bacteria, virus, and disease cannot live. This is good news for the CRC patient. Essential oils contain oxygenating molecules, which transport the nutrients to the cells of the body. Without oxygen, nutrients cannot be assimilated, leaving the body nutritionally depleted. They have been shown to increase oxygen by 21% in the human body. Essential oils also balance the pH of the body and maintain proper acid/alkaline balance.

New research work being done by Bruce Tianio is startling. Tianio identified the electrical frequency of essential oils and how different oils affect the body and its defense system. A frequency monitor meter (his invention) rates the electrical frequencies of natural and man-made substances. He believes all disease comes from an altered body frequency. [24] Tianio further says that applying these essential oils to various reflex points on the feet and elsewhere on the body assists in returning a normal frequency rate to various organs.

Dr. Gary Young discusses further the electrical impulses in relation to the body's health. He states that the normal electrical frequency for the human body is 66 hertz. [25] Illness is evidenced by a lower body frequency reading, ending at 25 hertz when death overtakes. When the frequency reading drops to 55 hertz, disease begins. The onset of CRC is even earlier, when the frequency reading drops to 57 hertz. Additional disease sets in when the frequency measures 58-60 hertz. The good news is that essential oils have frequencies ranging from 50 to 320 hertz. Applying these oils can beneficially raise frequencies within three seconds.

Not surprisingly, the known toxic substances of caffeine and nicotine lower electrical frequencies, allowing disease to commence. In the CRC patient, disease is already present, thus the consumption of caffeine beverages and the inhalation of cigarette smoke causes further degeneration. One research assistant who never drank coffee saw his electrical frequency drop from 66 to 58 hertz simply by holding a cup of coffee. When he took one sip, it slipped to 52 hertz. The same nonsmoker assistant held a cigarette and saw his frequency drop to 55 hertz. One puff plummeted his reading to 48 hertz. In taking no redemptive measures, it took three days for his frequency to return to 66 hertz. Conversely, in similar scenarios of reduced electrical frequency followed by the application of essential oils, his frequency returned to normal in three seconds. [26]

High-frequency essential oils such as the oils of cinnamon, cloves, tea tree, rosewood, and rose will all help to combat CRC. Rose, with a frequency of 210 hertz, is especially helpful.

Dr. Young also reports in *Together* that Dr. Radwan Faraq, from Cairo, Egypt, while lecturing in Utah, said that he has research demonstrating essential oils to have antifungal properties as well as therapeutic value. Dr. Faraq has received numerous awards for his research in essential oils and is credited with discovering the oxygenating molecule found in the oils. [27] The benefits of essential oils should be of interest to the individual seeking recovery from CRC.

Enemas and Colonics

A cleansing enema, or an infusion of fluid into the rectum, has been used for generations to relieve constipation. The rectum is the final eight to ten inches of the large intestine. Various substances can be used in an enema, such as mineral oil, castor oil, or coffee. All are designed to correct constipation and to cleanse the rectum. CRC patients can suffer from diarrhea and/or constipation. In the case of constipation, an enema can be a solution.

Enemas have been a part of conventional medicine for decades. Medical literature shows that coffee enemas were recommended by the Merck Manual from 1898 until 1977. (The Balchs also suggest that coffee enemas stimulate the liver to throw off toxins. [28]) After 1977, the section on enemas was omitted—not for medical reasons, but rather due to a space limitation. [29] Enemas are generally administered at home.

Enemas can be useful when herbal therapy has not been effective. Occasionally natural herbal preparations taken by mouth fail when abdominal bloating is severe. The patient's digestive acidic condition is so severe that it negates the herbal preparation. In these instances, Dr. Van Benschoten states that retention enemas are to be given twice daily. [30] He suggests that patients lie for ten to fifteen minutes on each side and then on their back in order to bathe the entire colon.

A colonic is an extended or more complete form of an enema. It is a gentle infusion of warm filtered water from the rectum to the cecum, offering greater cleansing and therapeutic benefits. A colon therapist generally administers the colonic. The Candida albicans overgrowth is greatly diminished through this direct method of colon cleansing.

Garlic

Garlic is another useful tool in the war against CRC, as shown in many studies and reports. A 1987 report in *Applied Environmental Microbiology* showed that garlic has strong antifungal properties which destroy the Candida albicans organism. [31]

Garlic is being shown to have many more health benefits than has previously been believed. Benjamin Lau, M.D., Ph.D., professor at California's Loma Linda University of Medicine, has specialized in microbiology and immunology for more than fifteen years and researched garlic in response to patients' requests. He cited another study, which took place in India, demonstrating the control of Candida albicans infection in chicks with the oral feeding of garlic. [32]

Famed health writer Jane Brody states in a *New York Times* article that the active ingredients in garlic "stimulate various immunological factors that may help the body combat cancer as well as stubborn fungal infections, like Candida albicans, a yeast that plagues millions." [33] The benefits of garlic are multiple.

Exercise

Dr. Mohamed A. Fahim found that those who exercise had higher levels of neurotransmitters. "Neurotransmitters help the brain communicate with muscles. With good communication and adequate levels of neurotransmitters, your brain can control your muscles." [34] A "foggy brain" or "spaciness," as described by many CRC patients, may be cleared by aerobic exercise.

"Increasing physical activity, particularly of light-to-moderate intensity, is appropriate to prevent disease and promote health," reports researcher Martha Slattery from the University of Utah Medical School. [35]

Oxygen

Oxygen is a gas that is essential to life. Hydrogen peroxide releases oxygen. It is a common drugstore antiseptic, at 3% strength. [36] Some CRC patients add this ingredient, at 35% strength (available in health food stores), to their bath in order to pull CRC toxins from the body, as well as to absorb oxygen. Typically, they start with one half cup and gradually increase to two cups.

OxyCleanse is an over-the-counter tablet formula that delivers oxygen in the form of magnesium peroxide. CRC patients are encouraged to use this as part of their treatment plan.

Water

For individuals recovering from CRC, it is especially important to drink plenty of pure, uncontaminated water. This will help soften stools and flush toxins from the system. Adding lemon will add an additional element of intestinal cleansing to the water. Eight glasses of water daily is optimal.

Conclusion

Using natural therapy for treating CRC can produce long-term results with no adverse side effects. Items such as herbs, herbal teas, vitamins, minerals, essential oils, enemas and colonics, garlic, hydrogen peroxide, and adequate water all help the CRC patient on the road to recovery.

Part Three
Research Findings

Chapter Eleven

Findings, Discussion, Conclusions, Recommendations

The Research Process

The research cited in this chapter was conducted and coordinated through my role as director of the East-West Clinic in White Bear Lake, Minnesota. A 37-item questionnaire was designed to provide feedback on questions relating to the management of Candida Related Complex (CRC). The questionnaire was designed to provide answers to several major questions:

1. Which treatment regimens (drugs, diet, nutritional therapies, etc.) were effective in reversing the symptoms of CRC?
2. Which *combination* of treatments were most effective?
3. Of the therapies that were effective, how long did it take before positive effects were felt; how long did it take before one fully recovered; and were there any adverse effects from these therapies?

Demographics

The sample was selected based on two criteria. First, all were people that were assessed as positive for CRC, either using the "Rate Yourself Test for Candidiasis" devised by John P. Trowbridge, M.D., and published in his book *The Yeast Syndrome*, or diagnosed by a medical doctor or a health practitioner other than a physician.

The second criterion required that respondents could claim that their symptoms were now reversed or significantly reduced. This conclusion was derived from a self-assessed comparison rating of symptoms before and after treatment and from a subjective rating of their overall health status.

Since the intent of the study was to determine treatment modalities that were effective in controlling CRC, it was necessary to seek out people who could claim that at the time they responded to the questionnaire, they had significantly fewer symptoms or were non-symptomatic. The group surveyed came from the pool of patients at the East West Clinic, and from the list of people who had purchased anti-fungal products and colon cleansers from a company in Minnesota that markets herbal and nutritional supplements for candidiasis.

Of the 70 questionnaires sent out to people who met the above criteria, 50 responded — a response rate of 71%. In this sample population, 76% were female and 24% male. Their ages ranged from 18 months to 82 years. Most of the population studied came from Minnesota (80%) and the remainder from other parts of the U.S. and one from Ecuador.

All the data presented are derived from the feedback offered by the respondents based on an analysis of their situation as it related to their experience with Candida Related Complex (CRC).

Health of Respondents

At the time they were surveyed, respondents rated their overall health according to these criteria:

11% Excellent health, not symptomatic at this time;
50% Symptoms are still there but very mild and manageable;
30% Symptoms come and go but could go for weeks without symptoms;
7% Symptoms come and go but could go for months without symptoms;
2% Symptoms come and go but could go for years without symptoms.

Diagnosis

When asked how they determined they had CRC, the 46 who answered this question, 41% claimed they were diagnosed by a physician (M.D.) in holistic practice, 53% by practitioners such as chiropractors, doctors of naturopathy and acupuncturists, and three respondents were self-diagnosed from reading books (6%).

Duration of Symptoms

Respondents were asked the length of time they suffered the symptoms of CRC before they were diagnosed (even though they didn't know what it was called then). Forty-five responded to this question, and their answers ranged from as few as six months to 41 years. Half of the respondents had suffered symptoms of CRC for six and a half years before being diagnosed. Twenty-five percent of those responding had CRC for more than ten years prior to being diagnosed.

Effect on Employment

At the time they were surveyed, 64% were currently employed and 16% of those employed worked full time. Most of the respondents (85%) claimed that they did not have to quit work because of their illness, and 15% claimed they could no longer sustain employment and had to go on a leave of absence or quit. Of those employed, 53% claimed they did not miss work because of this illness and 47% said they only missed work from time to time.

Expenses

Twenty-four people responded to the question on how much was spent on doctor's bills, hospitalizations, clinic visits, treatments, and purchase of products. A range of $450 to $98,000 was reported. Seventy-five percent claimed to have spent an average of $6,000 out-of-pocket (not covered by insurance). Less than half reported that insurance paid part of their expenses. The range of coverage was anywhere from 5 to 80%. Overall, for those who had partial coverage, reimbursement by insurance companies came to an average payment of 47.5%.

Product Effectiveness

Table A1—Number and Percentage of Respondents Using CRC-Related Products

Product	Number of Users	% Using CRC related products
Acidophilus	45	90%
Psyllium	45	90
Bentonite	43	86
Caprol	42	84
Garlic	27	54
Nystatin	27	54
Monistat	14	28
Nyzoral	13	26
Candida Extract	10	20
Diflucan	10	20
Caprystatin	7	14
Caprocin	6	12
Flagyl	5	10

From one to three respondents indicated use of the following products: Capronex, Chlorophyll, Citricidal, EDTA Chelation Therapy, Homeopathic Sepia and sulfur, hydrogen peroxide baths, Ketoconazole, lemonade with cayenne, Lotrimin, Nutrimin, Orithrush mouthwash, OxyCleanse, Pau D'Arco Extract, Sunrider Products, Terazol, and Yeast Away.

The above table shows the wide array of products that respondents in this study had used at one time or another during their recovery process. It is noted that the majority of people participating in this study used Acu-Trol products, i.e. the combination of acidophilus, psyllium, bentonite, and Caprol. Garlic and Nystatin were used by over one-half; Monistat and Nyzoral were used by one-fourth of the respondents.

The remainder of the products mentioned are listed in order to allow the reader to see the array of products available to the patient suffering from CRC.

After designating products which they had used, each respondent was asked to indicate what effect each product demonstrated. The respondent could choose to respond to as many statements as were appropriate. These statement options regarding their CRC condition were:

1. Improved significantly and improvement lasted.
2. Improved at first but symptoms came back after some time.
3. No change in symptoms.
4. Discontinued product because of side effects.
5. Discontinued because I am now well.
6. Continue to use this product.

Of the products reported as providing various levels of improvement, only the products used by at least 10 respondents are reviewed below.

Overview Of Product Effectiveness

In order to provide a general overview of the products' effectiveness, Table A2 was created as a way of combining the separate pieces of information reported in the subsequent pages.

This scale was created by formulating a ratio of positive-to-negative responses for each product. If the product was seen as providing "significant and lasting improvement" and if the user "discontinued its use because (the respondents were) well," the response was viewed as positive. Negative responses were: "improved at first but did not last, "no change in symptoms" and "discontinued because of side effects."

Table A2—Overview of Product Effectiveness Based on Positive Responses Divided by Negative Responses

Product	Number of Users	Overall Effectiveness
Caprol	42	1.92
Acidophilus	45	1.72
Bentonite	43	1.66
Psyllium	45	1.47
Diflucan	10	.33
Monistat	14	.30
Nystatin	27	.30
Nyzoral	13	.27
Garlic	27	.23
Candida Extract	10	.12

· A score of 1 indicates an equal ratio of positive to negative responses.
· A score of greater than one indicates a positive ratio.
· A score of less than one indicates a negative ratio.

According to the respondents, the four most effective products were Caprol, acidophilus, bentonite, and psyllium. These four products had positive effects that outweighed the negative effects.

The products that were least effective according to this scale are Candida extract, garlic, Nyzoral, Nystatin, Monistat, and Diflucan, with Candida extract being the least effective.

Table A3—Product Ranked by Respondents as Those that Caused Significant, Long-Lasting Improvement

Product	Number of Users	% Indicating Significant, Positive, Lasting Improvement
Bentonite	43	42
Psyllium	45	40
Caprol	42	40
Acidophilus	45	24
Diflucan	10	20
Nystatin	27	15
Nyzoral	13	15
Monistat	14	14
Garlic	27	11
Candida Extract	10	10

The three products which brought about the most significant, long-lasting improvement were bentonite (42%), psyllium (40%), and Caprol (40%), followed by acidophilus (24%) and Diflucan (20%). Nystatin and Nyzoral were rated effective, with long-lasting effects by only 15% and Candida extract was least effective (10%) compared to the rest of the nine products listed.

Table A4—Ranking of Products That Were Perceived to Bring Improvement at First, but Where Symptoms Came Back After Some Time

Product	Number of Users	% Indicating Improvement But With Recurrence
Monistat	14	42
Nystatin	27	41
Diflucan	10	30
psyllium	45	29
Caprol	42	26
Bentonite	43	23
Nyzoral	13	23
Candida Extract	10	20
Acidophilus	45	11
Garlic	27	11

Monistat (42%), Nystatin (41%), and Diflucan (30%) were ranked the highest out of ten products as those that gave only short-term improvement, and with symptoms recurring after some time.

This question of temporary improvement in some ways could reflect the fact that regardless of the product used, there is always some degree of recurrence. In addition, it should be noted that there are other variables other than product effectiveness that could cause a recurrence of symptoms, such as poor diet, stress, and lack of adequate rest.

The question was intended to identify the products which caused a recurrence, even while the respondent stayed with the recommended diet and was not suffering undue stress. It is not clear, however, whether respondents understood this and, therefore, the results of this particular question could reflect either situation.

Table—A5 Ranking of Products Which Were Perceived As Ones That Caused No Change in Symptoms

Product	Number of Users	% Indicating No Change in Symptoms
Candida Extract	10	40
Garlic	27	37
Nyzoral	13	30
Monistat	14	21
Nystatin	27	15
Acidophilus	45	11
Diflucan	10	10
Bentonite	43	7
Psyllium	45	7
Caprol	42	7

Candida extract (40%), garlic (37%), and Nyzoral (30%) were three products that were tried by our respondents, but ranked highest as ones that did not bring any change in symptoms. Bentonite, psyllium and Caprol (5-7%) ranked lowest, especially when viewed in light of the following table (A7). Most of the time these products were taken, they were effective in reversing symptoms.

Table A6—Ranking of Products Which Respondents Indicated Were Discontinued Because of Side Effects

Product	Number of Users	% Who Discontinued Due to Side Effects
Nyzoral	13	30
Candida Extract	10	20
Diflucan	10	20
Nystatin	27	19
Garlic	27	15
Monistat	14	7
Bentonite	43	5
Acidophilus	45	2
Psyllium	45	2
Caprol	42	0

Among the products used by respondents, Nyzoral, Candida extract, Diflucan, Nystatin, and garlic (15-30%) were discontinued most often because of side effects. Caprol, psyllium, bentonite, acidophilus, and Monistat (0-7%) were discontinued least often due to undesirable side effects.

Table A7—Ranking of Products Based on the Indication by Users That They Have Discontinued the Products Because They Are Well

Product	Number of Users	% Who Discontinued Because They Are Well
Caprol	42	24
Bentonite	43	23
psyllium	45	22
Acidophilus	45	18
Nyzoral	13	8
Garlic	27	7
Monistat	14	7
Nystatin	27	7
Candida Extract	10	0
Diflucan	10	0

The best products — ones that respondents took until they were well enough to discontinue their use — were Caprol, bentonite, psyllium, and acidophilus. Nearly a fourth of all respondents who have used one or a combination of these products could claim that, at some point, they achieved full recovery. Of the people in our study who used Diflucan and Candida extract, none could claim they got well enough to discontinue their usage. Of the 27 people who used Nystatin, only 7% could claim they were well.

It is to be noted that this survey was sent only to individuals who have recovered, and therefore these findings are significant to the extent that they reflect which products were most effective in bringing about long-lasting recovery.

When Improvement Was Perceived

The following table lists products that were rated as most effective in controlling CRC, the length of time it took for improvement to be perceived, and the total length of time it took for symptoms to completely clear.

Table A8—Ranking of Products Based on the Average Length (Months) of Time it Took For Improvement to be Perceived and Average Total Length of Time Until Symptoms Stabilized

Product	Number of Users	Length of Time (Months) It Took for Improvement to Be Perceived	Total Length of Time (Months) Until Stabilized
Psyllium	19	2.13	11.11
Bentonite	19	2.22	14.19
Acidophilus	17	2.79	16.11
Caprol	18	2.84	11.62
Nyzoral	14	3.30	13.30
Nystatin	11	7.95	23.46
Garlic	03	10.30	14.00

Table A8 data is given only where three or more respondents provided information.

Psyllium and bentonite were rated as providing the earliest signs of positive changes in symptoms. These indications came in slightly over two months (on average). Caprol, acidophilus, and Nyzoral showed improvement within approximately three months. Improvement with Nystatin and Garlic took from eight to ten months.

Thirty-five percent of those respondents who had taken either psyllium, bentonite, acidophilus, or Caprol claimed they felt relief within a week. While Caprol was viewed as taking slightly longer to take effect, both psyllium and Caprol were the only products where symptoms stabilized within one year. Nyzoral was seen as stabilizing symptoms earlier, on average in the 13th month, with bentonite, garlic, and acidophilus following closely with 14 to 16 months.

Nystatin was seen as bringing stabilization only after approximately two years.

With all the above products, it took a range of one month to three years for symptoms to stabilize to the point that respondents could discontinue usage. Approximately one fourth of them could claim they were stable within one to three months after using these products.

Table A9—Ranking of Products Based on Indication by Users that They Continue to Use These Products for Preventive Maintenance and When They Experience a Recurrence of Symptoms

Product	Number of Users	% Currently Using This Product
Acidophilus	45	49
Garlic	27	37
Psyllium	45	36
Caprol	42	33
Bentonite	43	30
Diflucan	10	20
Nyzoral	13	8
Monistat	14	7
Nystatin	13	7
Candida Extract	10	--

People recovering from CRC experience periods of remission and exacerbation. During periods of exacerbation (when symptoms) recur, they resume the use of anti-fungal agents and colon cleansers. This table reflects our respondent's choice for preventive maintenance as well as to control recurrences.

Acidophilus is the product of choice as ranked by 49% of our respondents, followed by garlic (37%), psyllium (36%), Caprol (33%), and bentonite (30%). Of the ten people that used Candida extract, none continued to take it for preventive maintenance. Very few (7-8%) used Nyzoral, Monistat, or Nystatin for this purpose.

Treatments Used as Part of Their Program for CRC

Acupuncture

Out of the 50 respondents, 32 (64%) used acupuncture as part of their treatment plan. As explained in previous chapters, the role of acupuncture in the treatments of CRC is to promote the body's ability to repair the damage done to it by the invasion of Candida.

Table A 10—The Favorable Effects the Respondents Claimed to Have Experienced with Acupuncture

Effects	% Who Used Acupuncture Claiming This Effect
Improved energy level	68
Ability to digest food better	62
Less bloatedness	56
Less sensitivity to substances	43
Fewer headaches	43
Fewer food cravings	31
Less binging	25

Other benefits mentioned by respondents were that it made it easier to relax, it relieved pain and inflammation, and that they just "felt better" overall.

A few of them (9%) reported having felt tired, cold, or sleepy for a day or two following the acupuncture session. One person reported getting slight hematomas (black and blue marks) at some acupuncture points; they disappeared in a few days. There were no other unfavorable side effects reported.

Respondents claim that they needed an average of 16 treatments to bring about significant improvement. Forty percent of them received these treatments on a weekly basis and 37% received treatments two to three times a week. About a third of them (31%) needed follow-up treatments to maintain the favorable effects, and these were done at an average frequency of every two weeks to once a month.

Forms of Treatment Used Other than Acupuncture

Respondents were asked to list other forms of treatment they used at one time or another while they were recovering from CRC. They were also asked to comment on the effectiveness of these treatments. The following table summarizes their responses to these questions.

Table A 11—Ranking of Other Forms of Treatment and Comments on Their Effectiveness

Type of Therapy	# of People Who Used Them	% With Positive Effect	% With Little or No Effect	% With Negative Effect
Chiropractic	26	57	43	0
Colonic Irrigation	12	91	9	0
Massage	10	100	--	--
Drugs (Antibiotics, Cortisone, etc.)	38	16	--	74

Other therapies used by one to four respondents and rated effective or helpful included: homeopathy, juice therapy, dental toxicology, sublingual drops, thyroid medication, and hair analysis.

Other therapies used by one to four respondents and rated effective or helpful included: homeopathy, juice therapy, dental toxicology, sublingual drops, thyroid medication, and hair analysis.

Half of the people in this study used chiropractic manipulation as part of their treatment plan for CRC. There is mixed reaction to this therapy: 57% of the respondents claimed it had a positive effect, and 43% said it had little or no effect on CRC.

Of the 12 people who used colonic irrigation, the vast majority (91%) said they had positive results and would recommend it to others.

Of the 38 people who listed drugs (such as antibiotics or cortisone) as a form of therapy, 74% noted a worsening of symptoms and 16% claimed they had a positive response. More research on this subject is recommended.

More research needs to be done as well to document the efficacy of chiropractic, colonic, and homeopathic treatments. The sample that responded to this segment of this questionnaire is too small to make any definitive conclusion.

Products Associated with Acu-Trol Program

Acu-Trol products refer to the combination of Caprol, bentonite, psyllium husks and seeds, and acidophilus. Of the 50 respondents, 43 (84%) used this combination of products. Since a large majority used these products, we wanted to elicit more information about their experience with these products. They were asked to comment on the length of time it took for this combination of products to take effect. Fifty-two percent claimed they felt relief within a few days, with another 42% stating they felt relief within one to three months after starting the program. The other 6% (or three people) said it took anywhere from five months to a year before they felt a change in their symptoms.

They were also asked to list favorable as well as unfavorable effects they experienced while taking the Caprol, acidophilus, bentonite, and psyllium products. Their responses were open-ended and they listed as many comments as they wanted.

Favorable Effects of Acu-Trol Products

The most frequently response was in relation to improved digestive functions.

Sixty-five percent reported feeling changes, such as less abdominal bloating and cramping, less gas, fewer bouts of diarrhea or constipation, lessened food cravings, and good bowel cleansing.

Thirty-two percent reported an increased energy level, less fatigue, fewer bouts of anxiety and depression, and increased mental alertness.

Thirty-one percent claimed to experience lessened sensitivity to food and other substances to which they were previously allergic. Comments under this category included less skin rashes, fewer allergies, sinuses more open, etc.

Twenty percent claimed to have lost a significant amount of weight. Some commented that they had tried weight loss programs before, but were not successful.

Eighteen percent indicated lessened joint and muscular pain.

Unfavorable Effects Experienced with Acu-Trol Products

There were fewer unfavorable effects listed than favorable ones.

Twenty-one percent reported having abdominal cramps, gas, and bloating initially. Other comments were single responses (and therefore not considered significant): too frequent bowel movements, dry skin, "die-off reaction" of fungi too strong, and products were too expensive.

Table A12—The Following Table Summarizes Responses Regarding the Overall Effectiveness of Acu-Trol Products

Overall Effect	% of Effectiveness
Significant change for the better	64%
Moderate positive effect	16
Mild positive effect	14
No effect at all	6

Combination of Treatments That Were Rated Most Effective

Respondents were asked to give their opinion on which combination of treatment regimens, protocols, etc., were most beneficial in controlling CRC.

In 60% of their responses, diet was mentioned as an essential part of the recovery process.

The combination most acclaimed (by 51% of the respondents) was adhering closely to the diet, using the fungicide Caprol (combined with acidophilus, bentonite, and psyllium), and using acupuncture treatments to repair the damages of Candida infestation.

Other combinations were mentioned by less than 10 people and, therefore, will not be considered significant. Some of these combinations are listed here, along with the number of people who used them with success.

Combination of Treatments Used With Success	Number of People
Diet, Acu-Trol, change in dental amalgams/ removal of mercury fillings	4
Diet, Acu-Trol, Nystatin	3
Diet, Acu-Trol, Chiropractic	3
Diet, Nystatin during crisis, Acu-Trol at end of crisis	2
Diet, Homeopathy	1
Diet, Nyzoral, Acu-Trol	1
Diet, Acu-Trol, acupuncture, hydrogen peroxide baths	1
Liquid combination of tea tree oil, Acu-Trol, lots of water	1

Combination of Treatments Reported to be Least Beneficial

"Use of fungicides without colon cleansers caused major die-off reactions and made me sick" is a comment repeated by 68% of the respondents. This comment explains why the use of detoxifiers like bentonite and bulking agents like psyllium to flush the dead fungus through the system more quickly makes so much sense.

"Antibiotics, cortisone shots, and creams caused a worsening of symptoms" was another comment mentioned repeatedly (by 40% of respondents).

Ongoing Maintenance

Diet Pattern Prior to Treatment

A comparison was made of diet patterns before the respondents became ill with CRC and after recovery was reached. The following is a summary of their responses:

- 50% noted that they ate "lots of sweets." Candies, chocolates, pastries, processed/refined foods, and breads made up a heavy portion of their daily food intake.
- 28% felt they had followed a fairly good diet before their illness.
- 10% said they only ate to survive; food made them sick.
- 9% reported drinking more than a normal amount of alcohol and caffeine, along with a poor diet.

Diet Pattern They Now Follow During/After Recovery.

- 35% say they eat mostly grains, a moderate amount of meat, fish, fresh vegetables, fruits, and minimal sugar.
- 30% say they eat whole foods, little or no sugar and practice a yeast-free and alcohol-free diet.
- 15% report eating a "normal diet," little sugar, yogurt, high fiber, and no coffee.
- 20% avoid meat completely, and have eliminated all greasy foods, sugar, and bread.

Overall, their eating pattern before they became ill was a classic junk food menu, rich in fat and sugar, low in fiber and nutrients. The upside of having had this illness seems to be that they learned how to eat properly. The experience of seeing patients through their recovery process allowed the researcher to watch this change in eating patterns. Their sense of wellness while they were sticking with the healthy diet became the primary motivator for eating right.

Exercise History and Current Practice

The responses to this question were mixed. Some exercised a lot, a few did moderate, regular exercise, and still fewer claimed they never exercised at all. The majority stopped most forms of exercise during the acute phase of their illness because of fatigue or the discomforts of the illness.

The current practice of the majority of those respondents who are now recovered includes a regular routine of exercise. Many mentioned walking, biking, tennis, aerobics, Nordic track, and swimming. Overall, the majority feel a heightened need to have an active life. They claim that this is a necessary part of their ongoing recovery program.

What Brings Symptoms Back?

An overwhelming majority (86%) claimed poor diet to be the most common reason for recurrences. This included eating sugar, yeast, alcohols, and excessive fruit. Stress came in second as a reason for exacerbation of symptoms, followed by antibiotics. Other culprits mentioned were: not enough or too much exercise; exposure to chemicals, smog, and fumes: not drinking enough water; and viral infections, such as colds or flu.

Programs Respondents Use for Maintenance

Thirty-seven patients volunteered to comment on this question. Sixty-six percent of them said they continue to use a modified Candida diet, restricting sugars and foods containing yeast. They also avoid alcohol and drink more fluids. Management of stress and getting enough rest were other items listed by many of the respondents.

A majority (60%) use fungicides and colon cleansers when symptoms begin to recur. A third use acupuncture as needed and a third also mentioned the use of ongoing multivitamin and multimineral supplementation. Other programs mentioned by a few include acidophilus, nystatin, homeopathic, chiropractic, colonics, regular exercise, and hydrogen peroxide baths.

Conclusion

In spite of the professional controversy surrounding the diagnosis of Candida Related Complex, as discussed in chapter five, it is a disease that is identifiable and can respond to appropriate therapy. However, it is a condition that is difficult to diagnose and takes many months to treat. In this study, most people affected by it were identified by practitioners other than a physician or were self-diagnosed (from reading books). Many people go for years without an appropriate diagnosis, visiting numerous doctors who treat them for the overt symptoms. In this study, 50% reported that they were ill for an average of six and a half years before their illness was recognized. Twenty-five percent suffered for ten years before they got help.

In our population, there were more women (76%) than men (24%), which supports other data that more women are affected by this illness than men. It can affect individuals of all ages. The causes are varied, but according to our data, a history of taking immunosuppressants such as antibiotics, corticosteroids, chemotherapy, and birth control pills strongly correlates with the development of CRC. Other factors that influence susceptibility are stress, poor diet and chronic illness.

Table A 13—Ten Products Most Commonly Used by People in the Study

Product Name	% who Used Product
Psyllium Cleanser	90
Acidophilus	90
Bentonite Magma	86
Caprol	84
Garlic	54
Nystatin	54
Monistat	28
Nyzoral	26
Candida Extract	20

Of the ten products, Caprol, bentonite, psyllium, and acidophilus were rated most effective. These products were rated effective because they gave significant improvement that was long lasting; they had fewer side effects and therefore people were able to continue using them. After a period of time, they were able to discontinue using the products because they had recovered.

The other products, garlic, Nystatin, Monistat, Nyzoral, and Candida extract, appear less effective in that they had more side effects and respondents could not continue using them. These products brought initial improvements, but symptoms came back after some time. For this group of products there is an indication that they brought no change in symptoms, i.e. no indication that the respondents were getting better.

Caprol, bentonite, acidophilus, and psyllium were referred to by respondents as the Acu-Trol program. More than one half of those who took these products claim they felt lasting relief within a few days and 42% claim they felt relief within two to three months. They took these products for an average of one year in order for symptoms to completely stabilize and so that they could reduce or stop their use.

The other products, Nyzoral, Nystatin, and garlic took even longer: three to ten months to feel a difference, and thirteen months to two years for the symptoms to stabilize.

The benefits of the Acu-Trol program were many compared to the reported unfavorable effects. The majority reported the changes in gastrointestinal functioning to be the most valued benefit. Changes such as less bloating, fewer bouts of diarrhea or constipation, lessened food cravings, and good bowel cleansing were listed. A third reported an increased energy level, less fatigue, fewer bouts of anxiety or depression, and increased mental alertness. Another third reported positive changes such as lessened sensitivity to food and other substances to which they were previously allergic.

The unfavorable effects noted by less than a third of the respondents involved having abdominal cramping, gas, and initial bloating. These were considered mild and not a reason to discontinue use of products.

The treatment rated most effective in repairing the effects of CRC was acupuncture, which was used by 64% of the respondents in the study. Those who used this form of treatment reported an improvement in energy level, ability to digest food, less bloating, less allergies and, in general, fewer symptoms. This form of treatment had relatively few side effects and brought long-term results.

Half of the respondents also used chiropractic manipulation, but with mixed response. About half of them claimed it was helpful and another 43% felt it had little or no effect on their symptoms.

Colonics were used by 24% of the respondents with very positive results, and this treatment was highly recommended by respondents as part of the treatment program for CRC. Massage was used by a few (20%) and also recommended.

Of the 38 people who used drugs (such as antibiotics and corticosteroids) 78% claimed these caused a worsening of symptoms and therefore discontinued their use. Only 16% claimed that these drugs helped the symptoms.

Diet that is free of sugar, yeast, fermented food, and alcohol was reported by 60% of our respondents as essential in controlling the symptoms of CRC. They also claimed that violating these restrictions brought back the symptoms and delayed their recovery process.

The combination of diet, fungicides, colon cleansers, and acupuncture was the treatment combination claimed by the majority (60%) to be most effective in combating the disease. They also strongly suggested that the use of fungicides without colon cleansers should not be practiced because they had "die-off" reactions. This comment explains why the use of detoxifiers (bentonite) and colon cleansers (psyllium and colonics) makes sense.

It is fair to conclude that CRC is difficult to treat and that it takes a long time for CRC symptoms to go away. If patients understood this at the outset, it will lessen their stress and give them encouragement to stay with the program recommendations.

There is strong support from our respondents of the need for an ongoing program of preventive maintenance. This includes attention to diet, regular exercise, stress management, and periodic use of acupuncture, fungicides, and colon cleansers. It is possible to go for months or years without symptoms once the overgrowth is back under control; however, these patients are more vulnerable to recurrences compared to the rest of the population (who have never experienced an overgrowth of fungi).

These findings are based on the responses of people who participated in the study, and who happened to have used the above-listed products at one time or another for the symptoms of CRC. It does not negate the possibility that there are products not listed here that may be effective in controlling CRC. However, for the benefit of those who are looking for effective ways to manage CRC, this study provides some answers that may be used as guidelines in the selection of products.

Discussion

At the East West Clinic, the combination of fungicide, colon cleansers, and acidophilus are used for the first two to three months in combination with diet and acupuncture. After the third month, if the patient is still symptomatic, or if they have experienced periods of relief but the symptoms still come and go, an alternate fungicide is given, such as grapefruit seed extract, garlic extract, or OxyCleanse. The practice of alternating fungicides every two to three months is based on the possibility that the fungus could have developed mutations that are resistant to one type of fungicide. Empirical observation showed that patients experienced "die-off" again for a short period of time after the new form of fungicide was introduced. This leads to the assumption that a new batch of fungi must have mutated and are now being killed by the alternate fungicide. This is a concept that has not been explored scientifically and would be recommended for further research.

Other Observations Concerning the Use of the Combination of Acupuncture, Diet, Fungicides, Colon Cleansers, and Acidophilus

The group that used acupuncture concurrently (once a week) with the special diet, fungicides, and colon cleansers recovered within a shorter period of time (two-three months) than those who used diet and fungicides/colon cleansers alone.

People who used fungicides but did not combine them with colon cleansers experienced more severe and more prolonged die-off phases. The conclusions one can make from this study is that whenever fungicides are used, they must be combined with colon cleansers and detoxifiers like psyllium seeds and liquid-bentonite in order to shorten and minimize the die-off phase. This way, the toxins secreted by the dead fungus are prevented from being absorbed into the system and are flushed through the gastrointestinal tract more quickly.

Based on the observation of the researcher, after three to four weeks following the introduction of the first form of fungicide, some patients developed rashes in different parts of the body. The rashes did not look the same on all patients. Some showed pinpoint red spots mixed with whitish spots that appeared in the neck and upper part of the chest. Some had these rashes in the legs. Sometimes they caused itching; however there were those that never developed itching. Other skin changes observed include an orangy discoloration of the skin of the face, arms, palms, and soles. This discoloration does not include the sclera (the white section of the eyes), nor is seen as generalized skin discoloration, hence very different from the type of jaundice coloration typical of hepatitis.

These skin changes were temporary and gradually faded in a few weeks to a few months. The researcher's assumption is that this can be explained by two possibilities. First, that the toxin secreted by the dead fungi is partly absorbed in the skin and is shown in this type of pigmentation, or second, that the live fungi try to get away from the GI tract where the active killing is happening and show up in the skin or other parts of the body. Often the patients used fungicides (like Caprol) topically and the itching was relieved. This observation is empirical and is recommended for further research.

The study of CRC is in its infancy, as it is a relatively new disease brought about by the discovery and use of antibiotics, corticosteroids, birth control pills, and other immunosuppressants. These drugs are not harmful by themselves, and they are necessary and lifesaving in many situations. It is the non-prudent use of these drugs that can lead to the development of other diseases like Candida Related Complex. CRC is a serious illness causing some annoying, debilitating, and persistent symptoms that can last for years. It is hoped that through the findings of research such as this, more people can become aware of how this disease is developed, how it is diagnosed and treated, and, most of all, that it is one disease that is preventable.

Part Four
Life After Candida Related Complex

Chapter Twelve

Continued Attention to Diet After CRC

After Candida Albican Systemic Overgrowth (CRC) is under control, there are certain precautions that must be taken in order to prevent the return of CRC. Continued attention to diet is one of these steps. Topics to be considered regarding diet include: knowledge and use of life-giving nutrients, such as carbohydrates (both simple and complex); the gradual reintroduction of CRC-restricted foods; food rotation diet; instant-nutrition juicing; immune-damaging foods; sugar and sugar substitutes and; and cooking methods.

Carbohydrates

Knowledge of carbohydrates is of prime importance to the former CRC patient — knowledge not easily acquired. Some say carbohydrates are good for you, others disagree. Long distance runners relate with glee their "carbo loading" binges just prior to a marathon. How can that be helpful if carbohydrates are bad for you? What is the truth behind carbohydrates?

The truth is carbohydrates come in two types, simple and complex. Simple carbohydrates are sugars and complex carbohydrates are starches. Ignorance of the distinction between the two types of carbohydrates and how they interact with fungi can result either in continued good health for the recovering CRC patient or a return of their dreaded symptoms.

Simple carbohydrates are to be reintroduced gradually and with caution. If simple carbohydrates are reintroduced too soon or if they are abused, CRC symptoms will return. Nutritional biochemist Jeffrey Bland mentions several studies which suggest that "simple carbohydrates, such as sugar, stimulate Candida growth." [1] Other health care professionals agree. Urologist James Balch, M.D., and nutritionist Phyllis Balch, C.N.C., clearly explain the dangers of simple carbohydrates. Sugar stimulates the pancreas to produce insulin, which the body needs to metabolize the sugar. Too much sugar intake overstimulates the pancreas, resulting in an overproduction of insulin. If sugar abuse is chronic, hypoglycemia (too little sugar in the blood) can result. Additionally, the pancreas wears out from overwork and diabetes can set in. Overstimulation of the pancreas can lead to the collapse of the adrenal glands, which affects our ability to handle stress. [2]

Additional research on sugar consumption reveals that sugar is also responsible for reducing the body's immunity as reported in *Beyond Antibiotics* by Drs. Michael Schmidt, Lendon Smith, and Keith Sehnert. [3] Sugar, for as long as five hours after consumption, they report, "significantly decreases the ability of white blood cells to engulf and destroy bacteria." The authors were reporting on work published in a 1973 issue of the *American Journal of Clinical Nutrition*. [4] Sugar consumption places a burden on the immune system, which in turn decreases the ability to fight bacteria. Continued sugar consumption will only prolong the CRC problem.

This team of writers goes on to state that the 1993 figure on the amount of sugar consumed per American annually is an alarming 130 pounds. This includes both refined and natural sugars. That is fourteen times more than 100 years ago. [5] Therefore, when reintroducing sugar to his or her diet, the recovering CRC patient is urged to use extreme caution. Returning to old eating habits too quickly will mean a return of familiar problematic symptoms.

On the other hand, complex carbohydrates are helpful in keeping CRC in check. The bulk from these foods provide fiber needed to stimulate the peristaltic action of the intestine. Peristalsis is the contraction of the intestine, occurring in waves, which propel the intestinal contents onward. As the fiber moves along the alimentary canal, James and Phyllis Balch state, it takes with it toxic substances that would, without the bulk of high fiber foods, become lodged in the intestine. Without high fiber foods, a toxic build-up occurs. [6] This, of course, is a perfect breeding ground for fungi and harmful bacteria. Foods containing complex carbohydrates include green vegetables, beans, whole grains, nuts, seeds, oat and rice bran, and fruits.

Gradual Reintroduction of CRC-Restricted Foods

Professor A. V. Constantini, director of the World Health Organization's Collaborating Center for Mycotoxins in Food, states in the newsletter *Mycotoxins in Human Health* that in order to remain free of CRC, patients should not feed the fungi living within the body and should strive to limit the growth of toxin-producing fungi in the gut. He suggests the following dietary guidelines to restrict CRC:

- Reduce the intake of foods contaminated with fungal toxins in stored grains, nuts, seeds, meats, and grain-fed animal products (meat, animal fats, butter, and whole milk). Because fermented foods encourage fungal growth, reduce intake of beer, wine, bread, and cheese.
- Eat fish, fish oils, garlic, onions, herbs, spices, soya, and yogurt. These foods inhibit the growth of fungi.
- Eat vegetables, especially green ones. Vegetable fiber decreases the toxicity of the fungal toxins which do enter our body. This food binds and prevents absorption of mycotoxins and aids in their removal by defecation. [7]

Another dedicated anti-fungal professional, John Trowbridge, M.D., outlines a very thorough dietary program for the CRC patient in four sequential phases called the Celebration of Healthy Eating Program. Phase 1 eliminates yeast-stimulating foods and is the most radical of the four phases. Phase 2 adds some fruits and grains. In the later phases, foods are reintroduced gradually, after progress has been made and improvement noticed. Phase 3 adds nuts and cheese. Phase 4 finally adds yeast-containing foods or foods with high sugar/carbohydrate content — foods that would dramatically encourage yeast growth in the immune-weakened person. These foods are sugars, including those made from beets, cane, corn, honey, maple, and molasses. [8]

In summary, the recovering CRC patient should eat a diet high in complex carbohydrates, including vegetables and meat, especially organic chicken, brown rice, and millet. Additionally, the consumption of live yogurt cultures containing acidophilus will reimplant beneficial bacteria in the gut. The use of hypoallergenic food supplements to avoid allergic reactions is recommended when restoring depleted vitamins and minerals.

Conversely, the recovering CRC patient should avoid simple carbohydrates, including all forms of sugar and overripe fruit. Also citrus and acid fruits (oranges, grapefruit, lemons, tomatoes, pineapples, and limes) should be reintroduced slowly, only twice weekly. These citrus and acid fruits are alkaline-forming; Candida albicans thrives on them. Also avoid dried fruits, because of the high probability of mold contamination. Also avoid alcohol (seven teaspoons of sugar in each shot of liquor), chocolate, fermented foods, aged cheeses (goat cheese or feta cheese is allowed), all grains containing gluten (wheat, oats, rye, and barley), ham, honey, nut butters, pickles, soy sauce, sprouts, vinegar (apple cider vinegar is allowed), and raw mushrooms (a fungus).

Food Rotation Diet Aids in Avoiding Allergies

Repeated overexposure to specific foods can bring on allergies. Allergies can cause multiple physical problems ranging from moderate to life threatening. A diet which rotates foods helps to prevent allergies from forming. Many CRC patients have allergies, so recovering CRC survivors should be aware of allergenic foods and avoid them. Many ex-CRC patients find that their allergies subside or disappear along with other CRC symptoms. Douglas Hunt, M.D., in his book on cravings gives some basic rules to follow to avoid allergies:

Basic Food Rotation Rules
1. Do not eat any food more than once every four days.
2. If a reaction occurs, it may come from another food in the same food group. Thus, patient may have to avoid that food group temporarily.
3. If patient reacts to many different foods, keep meals simple, with only one to three foods/food groups.
4. Moderate servings are preferable to large servings.
5. For 12 weeks, avoid any food that stimulates a reaction. After 12 weeks, don't use more than twice a week. [9]

Ironically, individuals with allergies crave the very foods to which they are allergic, thus CRC patients are strongly advised to avoid these problematic foods/food groups.

Instant-Nutrition Juicing

For the recovering CRC survivor, juicing can be an alternative when familiar cravings for sugar strike. Because cooked foods lose some of their nutrients, the juicing of raw and fresh foods are preferred, because vitamins and minerals remain intact in the juice. Jay Kordich, fondly nicknamed "The Juiceman" for his tireless promotion of juicing, gives seven basic rules for juicing.

Juicing Suggestions
1. Use organic produce that is pesticide- and chemical-free;
2. If organic is unavailable, wash available produce more thoroughly;
3. Peel oranges, grapefruit, and tangerines because of bitterness, but leave nutrition-rich white membrane;
4. Using more than a quarter of the juice from green leafy vegetables may produce gastric discomfort;
5. Bunch up leafy green vegetables prior to juicing. Use leaves of lettuce or cabbage to wrap sprouts;
6. Beginners should dilute juices by one quarter in order to become accustomed to the high concentration of nutrition
7. Drink juice immediately to avoid oxidation which occurs within a few minutes of juicing, and resulting in a loss of nutrients. [10]

By removing the fibers of vegetables and fruits through extraction (via a juicing machine), instant energy is provided. Nutrients are digested and assimilated in a matter of minutes, with a minimum of exertion from the digestive process. Of course, fiber is still necessary to stimulate the peristaltic action of the colon, but when a quick pickup is needed, juicing provides it. [11]

Juicing is good for recovering CRC patients and is healthy for all people.

Immune-Damaging Foods

A weakened immune system is an open invitation to the return of CRC. There are "seven sinister" food substances that Stuart Berger, a medical doctor and researcher in nutrition, feels most frequently create immune damage. The items, listed in order of most frequently to least frequently causing damage to the immune system are: cow's milk products; wheat; brewer's and baker's yeast; eggs; corn; soy products; and sugar. [12]

The adverse problems these foods cause are as follows. Cow's milk products, states Dr. Berger, can cause gastrointestinal problems with such symptoms as cramps, gas, bloating, diarrhea, constipation, and asthma. [13] Dr. Crook, a physician and allergist, also warns of the damage associated with the consumption of cow's milk products. He states that these products can also cause rhinitis, an inflammation of the mucous membrane of the nose. [14]

The next most commonly reactive substance is wheat. In *The Yeast Syndrome*, Dr. Trowbridge states that often severe diarrhea results from wheat consumption. [15] Also, other researchers suspect a possible relationship between wheat and multiple sclerosis. [16]

The next most frequent reactive foods are brewer's and baker's yeast. "Any yeast or yeast-containing food," says Dr. Trowbridge, "can feed or stimulate one's own internal yeast organisms." [17]

Next on the list of the "sinister seven" substances is eggs. Dr. Andrew Weil says eggs can be contaminated with bacteria. [18] He suggests that if eggs are eaten, cooking thoroughly is advised.

Next is corn. Dr. Trowbridge feels it is such a problem that he delays reintroduction of corn until the Phase 3.

After corn, soy products are next in frequency. Dr. Trowbridge states that soy products can be reintroduced in Phase 2, but that soy sauce should be delayed until Phase 4. [19]

Finally, Dr. Berger implicates cane sugar, which is commonly known to feed yeast, allowing them to proliferate. [20]

To support and foster a strong immune system, which can keep CRC in check, survivors are urged to beware of these "sinister seven" substances.

Sugar Substitutes

As already noted, sugar causes major problems for the CRC patient. Because so many people crave sugar, and because sugar feeds the yeast (which causes a rapid increase in Candida albicans or a resurgence of CRC), it is important to discuss sugar substitutes. CRC and ex-CRC patients must also be on the alert for hidden sugar in many foods, as well as vigilant about their daily use, or sporadic abuse, of sugar. There are several substitutes on the market. Some are good and some are just as problematic as sugar.

Aspartame, marketed under the brand names NutraSweet and Equal has gained in popularity since it was approved by the Food and Drug Administration in 1981. This sugar substitute is a combination of two amino acids, aspartic, and phenylalanine. Some leading natural health care professionals feel that occasional use of aspartame will do no harm. However, others do not agree. They feel that aspartame feeds the yeast in the same manner as sugar. An added element is that it cannot be used in baking. The Candida Research and Information Foundation reported that brain tumors and seizures have been linked to aspartame consumption. [21] Due to the conflicting reports on this product, it may be best to avoid its use.

Other sweeteners are honey, molasses, barley, rice malts, and vegetable glucose. The sugar substitute that seems the most satisfactory in regards sweetness, taste, and safety is stevia. It has thirty times the sweetening power of sugar. It comes from South America and the southwestern U.S. Stevia is water soluble, nonfermentable, leaves no aftertaste, and is not absorbed by the body. [22] When it first appeared on the market it was in a liquid form with a dark color and a strong licorice-like flavor. Later, a white version in a powdered form appeared and proved to be more readily accepted. This sugar substitute is delicious, safe, harmless, and has no side effects.

Cooking Methods

Since CRC patients are nutritionally deficient, it is important to use cooking methods that will retain as many nutrients as possible.

Steaming retains more nutrients than any other method of cooking. This method is especially good for cooking vegetables and fish.

Stir frying is a tasty, quick way to prepare a meal. Cook lightly for a short period, removing from heat when vegetables are still crunchy. Use lots of vegetables, adding a minimum amount of meat for seasoning. Use broth for the cooking liquid. Season with a variety of favorite, fresh herbs.

Broiling is quick way to cook without having to add fat (as in frying). Baking is another alternative, but does take additional time. Slow, crock pot cooking is yet another suggested method, popular for its plan-ahead ease in food preparation and because it retains nutrients. Charcoal grilling should be used with caution, avoiding excessive browning as foods cooked brown or dark may possibly cause cancer. [23] Refrain from frying foods, as this adds too much fat. Also refrain from boiling as this depletes the food of nutrients.

Microwave cooking poses the danger of leaking microwaves into the surrounding area. Andrew Weil, M.D., author of *Natural Health, Natural Medicine*, suggests a test for this hazard. "Hold a fluorescent light bulb in your hand and move it around the front of the oven while it is on. If the bulb lights or flickers, microwaves are leaking out." [24] If leakage is suspected, call a professional to check it out.

Conclusion

The recovering and recovered ex-CRC patient must continue to be vigilant about specific foods or else the nemesis can return. Most recovered CRC survivors have temporary set backs. The important fact to remember if and when set backs occur is to recognize what happened and return to proper eating habits. Knowledge of carbohydrates, both simple and complex, gradual reintroduction of certain foods as recovery takes place, food rotation, juicing for concentrated nutrition, foods that can weaken immune systems, sugar and sugar substitutes, and cooking methods, helps to achieve a wiser, healthier, eating pattern, and to keep CRC at bay.

Case Study Six

59-Year-Old Female Recovers From the Ravages of Candida

Almost 30 years ago, though I was only 29 years old, I was limping badly and dragging my right leg. A forward movement with that leg pained me so severely that I would audibly draw in a breath with each step, despite my resolve to grit my teeth and keep silent. I suffered from a pinched sciatic nerve.

I learned that tonsils are a vital part of one's immune system; mine had been removed when I was five! Next, at around age 16, I started to get a herpes-type sore on either nostril when I was under stress. As a young wife at 19, an occasional vaginal yeast infection, beginning with my first pregnancy, seemed minor. A year later, urinary tract infection (UTIs) started with the second pregnancy and required repeated rounds of antibiotics over the ensuing 14 years. In later years, I developed chronic, continuous cystitis — a burning at the bladder opening.

Realizing that conventional medicine wasn't able to resolve my UTIs, I felt compelled to look elsewhere for help with the sciatic nerve pain. This caused an extreme right foot sensitivity. I had to protect that foot at night from the pain of a rubbing sheet by sleeping with my left foot cupped over the right. A chiropractor helped, but only temporarily. After a few days of relief, the pain would return. It seemed as though my muscles were too weak to hold an adjustment. I was dependent on his treatment two or three times a week for 20 years.

Tracheitis and bronchitis began when I was 27, during the eighth month of a pregnancy. I was losing teeth at an alarming rate due to abscesses. At age 29, I was already sporting a partial plate. I also required a special toothpaste for sensitive teeth because mine painfully reacted to hot and cold. As further evidence of my discomfort, each morning I would noisily cough up phlegm.

I also had a lot of gas. No matter what I ate or how I ate, hungry or not, I was always burping — and not a nice quiet, ladylike burp either! A bloated distended stomach, as well as pain, accompanied the gas. I also experienced intermittent colitis. Gallbladder pain also troubled me occasionally. Sharp, racking pain signaled each attack.

Over the years, my weight was steadily increasing. I blamed my lack of self-control for not being able to master my sugar cravings. A sugar snack gave me a needed quick pick-me-up, but set up a craving for more and more sugar.

Additionally, my comfort zone was between 78 and 82 degrees. I began to dislike my elbows. If I scraped my fingernail across an elbow, a crusty film would come off. Likewise, my heels developed vertical cracks that snagged my nylons.

Often I remembered the Biblical verse in Psalms 22:17 "I can count every bone in my body." I could count my hand and foot bones by their throbbing. It finally dawned on me that this condition worsened after sugar consumption.

My fatigue was overwhelming. It felt like there was a hole in the bottom of my foot and all my energy drained out. Shortness of breath was also beginning to surface, especially when I had to climb steps or perform any other mild exertion.

I was unable to conceive after giving birth to stillborn twin girls (our 3rd and 4th children), my doctor placed the blame on an irregular menstrual cycle and prescribed birth control pills for a year. Later, I learned that oral contraceptives stimulate Candida growth.

After holding my own health for about fifteen years (still having sporadic infections, sciatic pain, sore teeth, etc., but not getting a whole lot worse), I entered menopause in my early 50s. That's when my health took a nose-dive again. Continuous infections, one after another, plagued me. The UTIs had escalated to the point that cystitis was always present except when I soaked in a warm bath. Sometimes I even fell asleep in the tub because it was the only place I was pain-free. The hot flashes I'd heard about for years were very real and particularly bothersome at night.

But, I guess God wasn't yet ready for me to become incapacitated with pain and illness. He sent me help. One week, my sister and I attended a seminar given by a naturopathic physician lecturing on auricular medicine (diagnosing and treating the body through the ear with acupuncture). On the third day when he lectured on hot flashes, he hit my buttons. Insensitively and insistently, I waved my hand and blurted out, "Can you help me?" He gently reminded me that he was in the middle of a lecture, but that he'd see me later. I wasn't about to leave (or let him leave) until he examined me.

Later, during the auricular exam, he could see that I was suffering from hot flashes. He assured me that he could successfully treat me; however, he warned me that the flashes would come back unless I took care of my root problem.

My underlying problem, he said, was chronic systemic candidiasis. He told me that my overgrowth of Candida was causing, not only hot flashes, but many other physical problems as well. These ailments would all go away or greatly subside, he continued, if I addressed the Candida.

The doctor treated my hot flashes and Candida with auricular acupuncture. He also told me that I needed to change my diet. No more sugar or breads, reduce red meat and increase vegetable intake. He looked at my sister and said he was sorry he didn't have time to examine and treat her, but that he was pretty sure she also had a problem with Candida.

Curiously, my sister and I had heard of Candida and a treatment for it only five days earlier, during an unplanned stop we made on the way to the auricular medicine seminar. A manufacturer of a Candida program explained CRC and his treatment program. We had told him that we were not interested in his product and parted company.

Now, I remembered this short visit with the manufacturer and was grateful for the free samples my sister had requested. These samples consisted of Caprol (olive oil with two anti-fungal acids), psyllium (an intestinal cleanser), bentonite (a detoxifier), and acidophilus (friendly bacteria). Arriving at my sister's home after the seminar, she said she would take the "stuff" if I would. So, we swigged the medicine at her kitchen sink and continued to take the treatment morning and evening.

After the first three days on the program, I experienced a heavy feeling in my arms and legs. It was a tremendous effort to lift my arms or walk. Later, I learned that this can be one result of killing off Candida and is called the die-off reaction.

Now for the good part of my story. When the leaden limb sensation left after four days, cystitis, which I'd had for the previous six months, was GONE. What a relief! Two weeks into the program, I realized that my old energy had returned to a level I hadn't felt for the past three decades. Within a month, my family realized that I had new energy. One day my 18-year-old daughter reminded me that, in a rash moment, I had promised to go Christmas shopping with her. Realizing that I'd had a nap that day (and that she had worked as a check-out clerk for eight hours at the corner convenience store), I felt I could tackle a short shopping excursion.

I must insert here that I was no shopper, because I would always get exhausted too quickly. As we entered yet another store three hours into our expedition, she moaned, "What's come over you, Mom? I'm tired. Let's go home." I delighted in chortling, "One more store, honey, just one more store," as she had so often said to me in the past.

At the same time, I noticed that I wasn't experiencing the UTIs. What a relief. Also I noticed I could go longer and longer between chiropractic visits, eventually ceasing altogether. It seemed my muscles strengthened because of the Candida treatment program and the adjustment finally held permanently.

I became so excited about my improvement in health that I wrote them down, lest I forget my former self and become ungrateful for my newfound health.

Additionally, the intestinal gas and burping problem decreased by about 95%. I didn't know where the bones in my hands and feet were anymore. The persistent cough was gone and the morning phlegm was no longer present.

After a few months, I realized that I could tolerate temperature variances just like other people, from 65 to 92 degrees. Formerly my comfort zone was from 78 to 82 degrees; this was an increase of 23 degrees.

One day, while applying makeup, I realized I no longer needed to use a cover-up for dark circles under my eyes.

Best of all, I could have an occasional sweet without setting up an uncontrollable urge to eat the entire contents of the cookie jar.

One pleasant surprise came after another. I liked my elbows and heels again. They were smooth, like a baby's; gone were the crustiness and cracks. My teeth no longer caused me discomfort; I didn't have to hold my lips shut in the cold weather and I could drink hot liquid without wincing.

I tried to get off the Caprol/bentonite/psyllium/acidophilus treatment program at four months and again at nine months, but both times (within two or three weeks) the herpes-type nose sore returned. This told me that I still had a Candida problem. I continued the program, all total, for fifteen months. The third time I stopped, my nose sore didn't return.

But then after a potluck dinner in our home, I nibbled on leftover sweets for three weeks until my nose symptoms returned. I then resumed the Candida treatment program for two more months.

In good health again, I was fine for the ensuing year and a half. But then a series of accidents bombarded me. A fall onto the edge of my sister's bathtub resulted in three cracked ribs. A month later, I stepped backward in a darkened restaurant without realizing there was a step down. I fell and jammed my bottom three vertebras. A week later, the car I was driving hit a deer and I sustained a whiplash injury. These three closely-spaced, painful accidents to my spinal column put so much stress on my immune system that yet another tooth abscessed and had to be pulled. The painful stress of these three spinal injuries caused a return of my nose sore and, thus, a necessary return to the Candida program. This time I needed four months of treatment to regain my health. Thankfully, for four years now, I've had my Candida under control.

As my health improved two years ago, I began walking. My husband recalls (I don't) that on my first attempt I could only go as far as the neighbor's house, about an 1/8 of a city block. I tired quickly, but I persisted.

After a year of walking up to a mile and a half, round-trip, the sciatic pain returned. Fortunately, I had already found Colet Lahoz, a wonderfully skilled acupuncturist. She had successfully treated me for an ulcer I developed just two weeks after my husband came down with his.

I sought her help in alleviating the returned sciatic pain. She observed that I had scar tissue surrounding the sciatic nerve and successfully treated it. Now I realized that there was help for old injuries that had ravaged my body during 35 years of Candida. Hesitantly at first, then confidently, finally almost gleefully, I mentioned to my acupuncturist the problem areas, one after another, as each surfaced over the ensuing months. These problems included sinus pain, tender breast scar tissue (caused by an infection while breast-feeding thirty years earlier), hearing loss and earwax build-up, lower back pain, and scarring on a kidney.

During one of the sessions, the acupuncturist placed several needles around my right jaw. Within a few days I felt a sore spot under my dental plate. As I've done before when this happened, I took it out for a few days, allowing the sore to heal. When I put it back three days later, it didn't fit. The bite was off. I had to go to the dentist to shave off some high spots so I could chew. Evidently, thirty years previously, when the dentist was working on my teeth, my jaw fell out of place. Not realizing this had happened, he constructed the partial plate to fit the misaligned jaw. That's probably how my temporomandibular jaw problem started.

I had another pleasant surprise coming. Over the years, my husband frequently urged me to stand straighter. But I couldn't seem to straighten up. I walked as if leaning into the wind. However, the more I walked and the more acupuncture treatments I had, the straighter I was able to stand. During one session, I asked the acupuncturist to needle my transverse colon. Later, while walking, a fascinating thing happened. Being now able to stand almost straight, I felt the urge to lift my rib case by standing even straighter. As I did this, I felt and seemed to hear a ripping sensation in my abdomen. It felt like part of my colon had been adhered to something in my abdomen and it just peeled off. Immediately, my shoulders reared back. Effortlessly, I now stood perfectly erect. This loosening of the colon allowed me to stand straight. That was a very strange experience.

That winter, on the return portion of my morning walk, I happened to notice my footprints I had made on the outbound portion of my jaunt. I stopped to stare. Both of my footprints were straight. Amazing! For decades my right foot veered outward, more to the right rather than straight ahead. Years ago, I had mentioned to my chiropractor the fact that my right foot turned out at an angle and not straight ahead. He said he realized my problem. It came from a misalignment of my hip, but there was nothing he could do about it. Now, apparently, acupuncture treatments had allowed my hip to return to a normal position and now my right foot pointed straight ahead.

I can't help but wonder if I had received acupuncture treatments at the time I started the Candida treatment program, if I would have been able to get the fungi under control much sooner.

It seemed that my body presented one area after another for healing. It was as if various body parts were waiting their turn to be taken care of. Poor body! I had made it wait so long for proper care and treatment. Now, nearing my sixth decade, I feel better than I did as a teenager. I'll save the rocking chair for later.

—Mary Johnson, St. Paul, Minnesota

Chapter Thirteen

Acupuncture Repairs Ravages of CRC

Acupuncture has long commanded respect as a pain reliever, but it is also effective in repairing, revitalizing, rebalancing, and stimulating organs and muscles. It is an excellent method to use in the recovery of Candida Related Complex (CRC). CRC, if unchecked, attacks one bodily system after another. This "domino effect" leads to damage of many physiological systems, one after the other. Not only does acupuncture address the acute, recent onset of physical problems, but it also treats chronic problems, including those organs damaged from embedded CRC.

In the book *Selfcare/Wellcare*, New York research professor and medical investigator Robert O. Becker is quoted as saying, "the prime function of the (acupuncture) system is that of sensing injury and effecting repair." [1] This age-old science is very beneficial in achieving recovery for the CRC sufferer who may have many organs in need of repair.

The World Health Organization (WHO) also considers acupuncture an appropriate treatment for many bodily ills which accompany CRC. These illnesses include: colds and flu, bronchitis, high blood pressure, ulcers, indigestion, hemorrhoids, diarrhea, constipation, earaches, dizziness, eczema, acne, headache, anxiety, depression, insomnia, infertility, premenstrual syndrome, pelvic inflammatory disease, gingivitis, irregular periods, and cramping. All of these symptoms have been experienced by CRC patients. WHO states that all of the above problems can be treated with acupuncture.

Energy

Acupuncture restores the body's vital energy force. Acupuncture also balances the energy flow between deficient and excessive levels. Energy levels are deficient because of tension. In this case, acupuncture could release tensions, which are blocking the flow of energy, thus allowing energy to once again circulate throughout the body via the meridians. This energy flow renews and repairs the CRC-damaged organs.

Conversely, sometimes there is an excess of energy and the patient is hyperactive. In this situation, acupuncture is used to moderate the energy flow. It is important to have the proper amount of energy flowing because then the body is able to repair itself.

Inflammation

Acupuncture treatments reduce inflammation which can still occasionally plague recovering CRC patients. As noted by a group of researchers headed by Dr. Sin at London's St. Bartholomew's Hospital in 1983, acupuncture is clinically effective in treating acute and chronic inflammatory disease. [2]

In a second study, Dr. Sin states that acupuncture actually halts a disease already in progress. He reports that, "acupuncture stimulation not only gives good symptomatic relief of inflammatory disease but also actually suppresses the underlying progress of the disease." [3] Acupuncture is of great benefit to the CRC recoverer because of its aid in fighting infections.

Pain

Acupuncture relieves pain from many sources, including the pain of a CRC-induced ulcer. "Acupuncture works," says Keith Sehnert, M.D., in his book *Selfcare/Wellcare*, "by causing the release of endorphins, natural opiates that bind to receptors and suppress pain signal transmission to the brain." [4]

A Czechoslovakian study reported in the *American Journal of Acupuncture* confirms this release of healing endorphins with acupuncture. In the study, ulcer patients suffered pain and indigestion commonly associated with an acute duodenal ulcer. The researchers saw a significant increase in the endorphins, while the patients were under treatment. [5] The endorphins regulate gastric and pancreatic secretion. Acupuncture treatments help the recovering CRC patient deal with the pain of a CRC-related ulcer.

Digestive System

The continuing health of the digestive system is of prime importance to the recovering CRC patient, since Candida albicans' stronghold is in this system. The digestive tract includes the mouth, esophagus, stomach, small and large intestines, liver, and pancreas.

The mouth is the site of the first recorded instance of CRC, some 2,500 years ago. Hippocrates wrote of the telltale white patches now known as thrush. This bothersome problem, which threatens some recovering CRC patients, can be healed with acupuncture.

The stomach digests food by secreting acids, hormones, and enzymes, which turn the food into chyme. Sometimes these digestive acids are out of balance — either too much or too little are produced. Acupuncture balances these digestive acids.

The liver metabolizes proteins, carbohydrates, and fats. During the metabolism process, food is transformed into usable elements for energy or growth. Impaired liver function promotes CRC-causing problems including chemical sensitivity, psoriasis, and PMS. The existence of these problems means that the liver is not filtering the blood properly. Two naturopathic doctors, Michael Murray and Joseph Pizzorno, in their book *Encyclopedia of Natural Medicine*, state that, "It is therefore important to support the liver before, during and after employing measures designed to destroy the yeast." [6] Acupuncture relieves congestion in the liver and stimulates its functioning.

The small intestine digests, absorbs, and transports food. The large intestine absorbs some elements, but it also stores and transports solid digested foods via the peristaltic action of the intestine. If ingested food substances are not transported in an efficient manner, then bacteria and fungi are allowed to grow in the stagnating material. Acupuncture aids the proper functioning of the intestines allowing for proper movement and elimination of fecal matter.

Digestive enzymes, produced by the pancreas, generally prevent the growth of CRC. If these enzymes are insufficient, Candida albicans can multiply and penetrate the intestinal wall. Acupuncture stimulates the pancreas to produce the enzymes necessary to digest food. The pancreas also produces insulin. Insulin, when secreted into the bloodstream, allows the metabolism and utilization of sugar, an added benefit for CRC patients. The pancreas can under produce insulin, resulting in diabetes mellitus or hypoglycemia. Acupuncture enables metabolism to function more efficiently. It also balances the production of the insulin hormone.

If Candida albicans is destroyed in the intestinal tract and not allowed to leak into the bloodstream, then CRC will not recur. Acupuncture heals the digestive system, which prevents a CRC recurrence.

Circulation

Circulation is the passage of the blood from the heart to all parts of the body. Blood transports nutrients and then returns from the outlying tissues to the heart again, carrying away waste products in the process. Often CRC patients experience sluggish circulation manifested by cold hands and feet. Acupuncture stimulates circulation.

The lymphatic system, which includes the spleen, thymus, and lymph nodes, is also part of the circulation system of the body. Acupuncture balances and restores the lymphatic system.

Urinary Tract

The urinary system includes the kidneys, ureters, and bladder. This system excretes liquid waste. When this is a weakness in the system, it becomes a haven for candida albicans once the patient develops systemic candidiasis. During the recovery process, acupuncture can heal scar tissue that has resulted from these many CRC-induced urinary tract infections. It also restores and tones the urinary tract keeping it in balance.

Muscular System

The entire muscular system can be invaded by CRC. Unfortunately, the heart, the most important muscle, can be a prime target. "Significantly," writes Rupert Beebe, author of Candida Yeast Infection: The Silent Killer, "disseminated (spreading) Candida infection has a particular affinity for heart valves." [7] Often the entire muscular system is weakened by CRC. Fortunately, ridding the body of CRC will allow this system to recuperate. Acupuncture can help in this process and heal these affected parts at a quicker pace.

Lungs

CRC can also invade the upper respiratory system. Chronic bronchitis and repeated bouts of pneumonia can damage the bronchial tubes and lungs. Chronic asthma, colds, and sinusitis that does respond to other forms of therapy is also an indication that CRC is present.

Acupuncture can decongest, tone, and repair these damaged upper respiratory organs.

Brain

The brain can also be significantly affected by CRC. Many patients describe their mental symptoms as fogginess, spaciness, inability to concentrate, absence of mental clarity, and disorientation. Mood swings can also be an effect of CRC. Because of these CRC-related symptoms, the patients often experience mental anguish and are fearful and worried.

The WHO lists anxiety, depression, stress, and insomnia as conditions for which acupuncture is considered appropriate. These conditions can all, as seen above, be CRC-related. Thus, acupuncture helps heal the ravages caused by impaired brain function.

Adrenal Glands

The adrenal glands, part of the endocrine system, also need acupuncture support following CRC. These glands produce cortisone and adrenaline. They regulate the salt/water balance of the body, the metabolism of carbohydrates, and the regulation of blood sugar. The adrenal glands also produce the sex hormones needed for the ovaries and testes. CRC can adversely affect the adrenals. Acupuncture can stimulate these glands to produce the natural type of cortisone. CRC-induced stress puts a tremendous burden on the adrenals; acupuncture can help to relieve that tension and stress.

Conclusion

In summary, CRC is able to invade any part of the body, injuring tissues as it progresses. During CRC recovery, acupuncture — by healing scar tissue, balancing the systems, revitalizing, toning, and repairing the damaged part of the body — is an important element in the healing process.

Chapter Fourteen

Steps to Prevent Recurrence of CRC

Certain steps must be taken by the recovering Candida Related Complex (CRC) patient. If these steps are not followed, CRC will return. These steps include continued attention to diet (as discussed in an earlier chapter), as well as the avoidance of antibiotics, oral contraceptives, stress, and harmful chemicals. Keeping the colon clean, maintaining a positive attitude, and regular exercise will also help in recovery. It is important that the recovering CRC patient also understand and expect retracing (when old symptoms are reactivated and resolved during the healing process).

In fact, the former CRC patient must avoid whatever it was that initially caused him or her to fall victim to this illness in the first place and should take specific steps which can hasten the healing process.

Prescription Drugs vs. Natural Medicine

Since a history of repeated use of antibiotics, corticosteroids, and/or immunosuppressant drugs is one of the main causes of CRC, preventing a return of CRC means avoiding these drugs.

There is a difference between natural and synthetic (prescription) medications. Synthesis means the formation of complex substances out of a combination of simple substances. In making synthetic drugs, the pharmaceutical companies extract active principles from plants; these ingredients are more powerful, but, because they do not contain the whole plant, they lack the natural safeguards present in the original plant.

There are a number of natural medicines that can be used as an alternative to prescription drugs. A high priority is Echinacea, writes Andrew Weil, M.D., in *Natural Health, Natural Medicine*. He states that Echinacea is a natural antibiotic, antiviral, and antibacterial and an immune-system enhancer. It comes in tinctures, capsules, tablets, and extracts. Echinacea causes a numbing sensation when held in the mouth for a few minutes. Dr. Weil suggests using this simple test in order to insure that the intended Echinacea is an effective product. This product loses its effectiveness upon continuous use. To avoid this, use it for 7 to 10 days at a time and use alternate types like Goldenseal if needed. [1]

Another natural product to use in place of prescription drugs is goldenseal. This is also available in many forms. Goldenseal tones the digestive system and has a reputation, says Dr. Weil, as a blood purifier. "I sometimes recommend it (goldenseal)," he says, "to people who are debilitated, have weak digestive systems, or are susceptible to recurrent infections." Dr. Weil also suggests using goldenseal topically for wound healing, as a disinfectant, and for scab promotion. [2]

A Clean Colon

Diverticulum is a sac arising from the colon wall. The presence of many small sacs or pouches projecting outward from the wall of the colon is called diverticulosis. Diverticulitis is an inflammation of a diverticulum of the bowel. Lack of fiber or roughage in the diet is believed to cause this condition. Many CRC patients and survivors have diverticulosis. Of special interest to the CRC survivor is the fact that Candida albicans live and multiply in the undigested food lodged in these sacs. So, it is of paramount importance that these sacs be cleaned out and stay clean. If the breeding ground for Candida albicans is destroyed, then CRC will disappear.

It takes a great deal of time to accomplish this cleaning task — often many months. Fiber in the diet will accomplish this task. Fiber is the portion of food that passes through the intestinal tract without being absorbed. Fibers come in seven categories, state James and Phyllis Balch in *Prescription for Nutritional Healing*: pectin, bran, cellulose, hemicellulose, lignin, gums, and mucilages. Pectin, cellulose, hemicellulose, and lignin are found in certain vegetables, fruits, whole grains, and Brazil nuts. Bran from rice and oats is the broken coating of the seed or cereal grain. Gums and mucilages are found in oatmeal, dried beans, and seeds. [3] Psyllium seeds and husks mentioned in an earlier chapter fall in this category. It is clear then that CRC survivors are urged to eat lots of high fiber foods such as vegetables, fruits, whole grains, fresh nuts and seeds, not stored nuts and seeds as they can be moldy.

Stress

People react to stress in an individual manner. When the level of stress reaches a certain intensity, it can begin to damage the immune system. A damaged immune system cannot fight off an attempted return of CRC. This level can vary from individual to individual. When damage occurs, the stress causes an excessive increase in the output of the adrenal gland hormones, write Michael Murray and Joseph Pizzorno in an *Encyclopedia of Natural Medicine*. [4] The damage occurs when these excessive hormones inhibit white blood cells (which fight infection) and cause the thymus (part of the immune system) to shrink, thus leading to a weakened immune system.

There are five ways to control stress, writes Keith Sehnert, M.D., author of *Selfcare/Wellcare*:

- Change work/social environment
- Understand emotions
- Learn ways to relieve stress
- Take care of the body
- Provide for spiritual needs [5]

Knowing how stress adversely affects the immune system and taking positive steps to control stress will help this system function at top efficiency and ward off a return of CRC.

Attitude

Attitude influences behavior; behavior influences health. A positive attitude influences behavior positively. A negative attitude influences behavior negatively. Changing from negative to positive can be accomplished by thinking positive thoughts and refusing to dwell on the negative. The more often one dwells on the positive, the more able one is to feel positive. This sounds ridiculous, but positive thinking is actually part of the healing process. When negative thoughts crowd the mind, these should be refused. Instead, the recovering CRC patient is urged to search until one positive thought, no matter how insignificant, appears and dwell on that thought. Gradually, more positive thoughts will emerge. This is the healing process from negative to positive — sadness to cheerfulness.

Along with a deliberate mental intention to choose positive thoughts, it is important to support the physical body with remedial nutritional supplements. A negative mental state is a condition that can result from nutritional deficiency. In fact, changes in mood are often the first sign of a nutritional deficiency. These mood changes include depression, memory loss, anxiety, and irritability. [6] The CRC recoverers need to monitor their nutrition habits and to quite possibly take nutritional supplements to help ward off the return of CRC.

Oral Contraceptives

There are several reasons why oral contraceptives should be avoided as a form of birth control. Ross Trattler, M.D., in his book *Better Health Through Natural Healing*, shares his insights on this matter. The most detrimental side effect of the pill, he states, is that it "provides the ideal environment for vaginal (yeast) infection." [7]

John Trowbridge, M.D., in his book *The Yeast Syndrome*, elaborates on this point:

> The attachment of steroids in birth control pills to receptor sites on C. albicans might 'feed' the yeast a desired molecule. Thus, oral contraceptives probably promote Candida colony growth through a direct and unavoidable mechanism . . . A woman swallowing her daily hormone-containing birth control pill might therefore be helping to meet the metabolic needs of Candida albicans. Her own cells are absorbing the progesterone from the pill. In penetrating human cells while searching for nutrients, the fungus is likely also to be stimulated by the steroids found within — resulting in more vigorous symptoms of the yeast syndrome. [8]

Intake of the oral contraceptive pill provides nutrition for the fungi, allowing them to flourish. The steroids in human cells also stimulate the fungi.

Oral contraceptive pills can lead to additional negative consequences, Dr. Trattler states. Use of these pills can cause fluid retention, depletes many of the B complex vitamins, especially B6, [9] interferes with carbohydrate metabolism, [10] doubles the user's chances of gallstones, [11] and causes Vitamin E deficiency. [12]

Furthermore, Dr. Trattler states that oral contraceptives upset the entire hormonal balance. After discontinuing their use, many women "fail to regain normal menstrual flow for varying periods of months to several years." [13]

Environment

Substances in the environment will affect the progress of CRC healing. Limiting exposure to reactive materials, such as foreign chemicals and molds, will help quicken and maintain recovery.

William Crook (who himself reacts to printing ink) cites numerous other substances that can trigger reactions: perfumes, insecticides, petrochemicals (automobile exhaust), household cleaners, tobacco, [14] formaldehyde in glue, chemicals added to drinking water, aerosol chemicals, drugs, [15] rubber, plastics, synthetic fabrics, dyes in clothing, waxes/polishers, paints, and cosmetics. [16]

Dr. Crook suggests that environmental reactions can include "burning eyes, stuffy nose, itching, tingling, headache, muscle and joint pain, and all sorts of unusual mental and nervous symptoms." [17]

Molds in closets, rugs, basements, or any other humid, moist environment can cause an aggravation of CRC-related symptoms, such as nasal drainage and extreme fatigue.

After CRC is subdued, chemical sensitivities will often improve; however, during the recovery period, it is best to avoid exposure.

Exercise

"Exercise stimulates adrenal activity and is useful in moderation," states Larry Wilson, M.D., author of *Nutritional Balancing and Hair Mineral Analysis*. [18] Moderate exercise helps the adrenals function as designed. Normal adrenal activity includes cortisone and adrenaline production, fluid balancing, carbohydrate metabolism, and blood sugar regulating.

Marcia Starck in her book *The Complete Handbook of Natural Healing* agrees with Dr. Wilson and adds other benefits of exercise, such as improved metabolism, digestion, circulation, and all other bodily processes. Starck claims that "physical exercise is one of the most important ingredients in maintaining health and balance." Additionally, she feels that exercise helps rid the body of toxins and aids it in assimilating minerals. [19]

Starck suggests that exercise can take the form of running, jogging, dancing, walking or sports such as tennis, basketball, racquetball, golf, and swimming. She also suggests that we view utilizing nature trails and participating in lake and river sports as ways of appreciating nature. [20]

The CRC survivor can speed recovery by participating in one or more forms of exercise.

Retracing

Retracing, also called healing reactions or healing crisis, Dr. Wilson states, is the situation when old symptoms or conditions are reactivated and resolved during the process of healing. [21]

Commonly, chronic infections or poorly healed wounds, injuries, or scars will go through a retracing process when using natural healing programs, becoming acute for a few days as the disease process is resolved. Emotional retracing also occurs as old feelings or memories are brought to consciousness and released. [22]

Some who are in the process of recovery mistakenly feel they are experiencing an illness when in fact it is the retracing process.

Dr. Wilson feels there are several changes that take place during the healing of not only physical ills, but also emotional and psychological ones as well. During the healing process, mind, body, and emotions are involved. This healing process can cause physical changes, such as reactivation of previous illnesses to a lesser degree.

For example, a chronic condition can suddenly flare up and become acute. This condition can also be called a completion reaction, states Dr. Wilson, "because the body is completing an effort which it previously was unable to carry to a resolution." For example, scars can itch, ache, or swell for a day or two. This healing crisis can also cause slowed metabolism and toxic waste elimination. Past traumas can finally be resolved, releasing stored emotions. [23]

Retracing situations are usually of short duration and should be accomplished by rest and reassurance. Dr. Wilson suggests that if a healing crisis is accompanied by infections, that vitamins A and C are helpful. If a toxic metal elimination is occurring, use hot Epsom salts or sauna baths, coffee enemas, and/or colonic irrigations. When an emotional retracing happens, a strong, friendly shoulder is helpful. If fatigue accompanies retracing, extra B vitamins are recommended. Finally, if the crisis involves anxiety and nervousness, Dr. Wilson suggests extra calcium, magnesium, zinc, choline, and inositol. [24] Acupuncture can also alleviate retracing situations and can bring about a more thorough healing.

Conclusion

There are certain substances and situations that the recovering CRC patient must avoid, such as prescription drugs, stress, oral contraceptives, and toxins in the environment. Conversely, there are certain beneficial situations and activities that will aid in recovery, such as a clean colon, positive attitude, exercise, proper nutrition, and a healthy energy balance. Finally, recovering CRC patients will find that knowledge of retracing is especially helpful.

Notes

Chapter One

1. Susan Cruzan, "Yeast Treatment." *Food and Drug Administration Press Office* (3 December 1990).

2. W. Krause, H. Matheis, and K. Wulf, "Fugemia and Funguria after Oral Administration of Candida Albicans," *Lancet* (22 March 1969): 598-599.

3. A. V. Constantini, "Definition of Mycotoxins," *Human Health Newsletter* 1, no. 6 (January 1994): 1.

4. Orian C. Truss, "Metabolic Abnormalities in Patients with Chronic Candidiasis: The Acetaldehyde Hypothesis," *Journal of Orthomolecular Psychiatry* 13, no. 2 (1984): 66-93.

Chapter Two

1. Orian C. Truss, "Metabolic Abnormalities in Patients with Chronic Candidiasis: The Acetaldehyde Hypothesis," *Journal of Orthomolecular Psychiatry* 13, no. 2 (1984): 66-93.

2. Excerpted from information published in *The New England Journal of Medicine*. Hawthorn Walsh, et al., "Detection of Circulating Candida Enolase by Immunoassay in Patients with Cancer and Invasive Candidiasis," 324, no. 15 (11 April 1991): 1026-1031. Massachusetts Medical Society. All rights reserved.

3. Excerpted from information published in *The New England Journal of Medicine*. John E. Edwards, "Invasive Candida Infections: Evolution of a Fungal Pathogen," 324, no. 15 (11 April 1991): 1060-1062. Massachusetts Medical Society. All rights reserved.

4. Douglas Hunt, "How Fungus Can Cause Cravings," in *No More Cravings* (New York, New York: Warner Books, 1987), 110-129.

Chapter Three

1. Rupert Beebe, *Candida Yeast Infection: The Silent Killer* (Vancouver: Healthology Association, 1988), 45.

2. Orian C. Truss, "Metabolic Abnormalities in Patients with Chronic Candidiasis: The Acetaldehyde Hypothesis," *Journal of Orthomolecular Psychiatry* 13, no. 2 (1984): 66-93.

3. Excerpted from information published in *The New England Journal of Medicine*. John E. Edwards, "Invasive Candida Infections: Evolution of a Fungal Pathogen," 324, no. 15 (11 April 1991): 1060-1062. Massachusetts Medical Society. All rights reserved.

4. Excerpted from information published in *The New England Journal of Medicine*. Hawthorn Walsh, et al., "Detection of Circulating Candida Enolase by Immunoassay in Patients with Cancer and Invasive Candidiasis," 324, no. 15 (11 April 1991): 1026. Massachusetts Medical Society. All rights reserved.

5. Betty B. Jorgensen, "Baker's Yeast Allergy in Candidiasis Patients," *Journal of Advancement in Medicine* 7, no. 1 (Spring 1994): 43-49.

6. John Parks Trowbridge and Morton Walker, *The Yeast Syndrome* (New York, New York: Bantam Books, 1986): 100.

7. Douglas Hunt, *No More Cravings* (New York, New York: Warner Books, 1987): 148.

8. William G. Crook, *The Yeast Connection* (Jackson, Tennessee: Professional Books, 1991): 27-28.

Chapter Four

1. Leo Galland, "Science and the Candida-Related Complex (CRC)," *Candida Update Syllabus*, International Health Foundation (17 September 1988): 21.

2. Plumlee, Larry. *Plumlee Compilation*. Human Ecology Action League. February, 1980. p. 3.

3. James Balch and Phyllis Balch, "Allergies." *Prescription for Nutritional Healing* (Garden City Park, New York: Avery Publishing, 1990): 78.

4. Orian C. Truss. "Metabolic Abnormalities in Patients with Chronic Candidiasis: The Acetaldehyde Hypothesis," *Journal of Orthomolecular Psychiatry* 13, no. 2 (1984): 66-93

5. A. V. Constantini, "Crohn's Disease: The Fungal-Mycotoxin Aspects of Intestinal Findings and Extraintestinal-Related Diseases," *Mycotoxins in Human Health Newsletter* 1, no. 3 (March 1994): 1.

6. A. V. Constantini, "The Fungal/Mycotoxin Connections: Autoimmune Diseases, Malignancies, Atherosclerosis, Hyperlipidemias, and Gout," (transcript of 28th Annual Meeting of New Horizons in Chemical Sensitivities: State of the Art Diagnosis and Treatment, October, 1993): 3031.

7. Sehnert, Struve, Komoto and Fosse. "An Evaluation of Self-Administered Questionnaires as an Aid in Diagnosis of Candida-Related-Complex," *Journal of Advancement in Medicine* 3, no. 2 (Summer 1990).

8. John Parks Trowbridge and Morton Walker, *The Yeast Syndrome* (New York, New York: Bantam Books, 1986), 100, 102.

9. William G. Crook, "Dr. Crook's Yeast Questionnaire and Score Sheet," quoted in John Parks Trowbridge and Morton Walker, *The Yeast Syndrome* (New York, New York: Bantam Books, 1986), 101, 102.

Chapter Five

1. Orian C. Truss, "Tissue Injury Induced By Candida Albicans: Mental and Neurologic Manifestations," *Journal of Orthomolecular Psychiatry* 7, no. 1 (1978): 17-37.

2. Orian C. Truss, "Metabolic Abnormalities in Patients with Chronic Candidiasis: The Acetaldehyde Hypothesis," *Journal of Orthomolecular Medicine* 13, no. 2 (1984): 66-93.

3. Chai Anderson et al., "Candidiasis Hypersensitivity Syndrome," *Journal of Allergy Clinical Immunology* 78, no. 2 (1986): 271-73.

4. Council on Scientific Affairs, "In Vivo Diagnostic Testing and Immunotherapy for Allergy" *Journal of the American Medical Association* 258, no. 11 (1987): 1505-08.

5. "Top Ten Health Frauds," *FDA Consumer*, October 1989, 29-31.

6. Gary Holt and Joanne Morici, "Hazardous Health 'Cures,'" *Family Circle* 5 May 1990, 27-30.

7. James P. Carter, *Racketeering in Medicine: The Suppression of Alternatives* (Norfolk, Virginia: Hampton Roads Publishing Company, 1992), cited in *Second Opinion.* (October 1993): 3.

8. Elizabeth Neus, "UC wins grant to study fungal infections," *Cincinnati Enquirer*, 24 January 1990.

9. P. N. Kasckin, "Some Aspects of the Candidosis Problem," *Mycopathologia et Mycologia* 53, (1974): 173-181.

10. Excerpted from information published in *The New England Journal of Medicine*. Eisenberg, Kessler, Foster, et al., "Unconventional Medicine in the United States: Prevalence, Cost, and Patterns of Use," 328, no. 4 (28 January 1993): 246-52. Massachusetts Medical Society. All rights reserved.

11. "It's the Law: There is an Office of Alternative Medicine," *AM Newsletter* 1, no. 1 (September 1993): 1.

Chapter Six

1. Leo Galland and Stephen Barrie, "Intestinal Dysbiosis and the Causes of Disease," *Journal of Advancement in Medicine* 6, no. 2 (Summer 1993): 67-81.

2. A. Huniset, J. Howard, and S. Davis, "Gut Fermentation (or the Auto-Brewery) Syndrome," *Journal of Nutritional Medicine* 1 (1990): 33-38.

3. Galland.

4. Slutsky, Buffo, and Soll, "High-Frequency Switching of Colony Morphology in Candida Albicans," *Science* 230 (8 November 1985): 666-69.

5. John Travis et al., "Frontiers in Biotechnology: Resistance to Antibiotics," *Science* 264 (15 April 1994), 360-93.

6. B. D. Colen, "Am I Going to Die?" *Ladies Home Journal*, October 1992, 90-94.

7. Paul Raeburn, "Medical Experts Fear Drug-Resistant Bacteria," Associated Press, 20 February 1994, in Fort Worth Star-Telegram, 1, 12.

8. Terence Monmaney, "Marshall's Hunch," *The New Yorker*, 20 September 1993, 64-72.

9. Douglas Piper, "Bacteria, Gastritis, Acid Hyposecretion, and Peptic Ulcer," *Medical Journal of Australia* 142 (15 April 1985): 431.

10. James A. Jackson, Ronald E. Hunninghake, and Neil Riordan, "Illness and Intestinal Parasites," *Journal of Orthomolecular Medicine* 7, no. 4 (1992): 202.

11. Ibid.

12. Leo Galland, "Diagnosing Amoeba by Rectal Swab," *Townsend Letter for Doctors* 65 (December 1989): 1-2.

13. William G. Crook, *Chronic Fatigue Syndrome and the Yeast Connection* (Jackson, Tennessee: Professional Books, 1992), 318-19.

14. Marian Segal, "Parasitic Evaders and the Reluctant Human Host," *FDA Consumer* (July/August 1993): 7-13.

15. Madeleine J. Nash, "The Waterworks Flu," *Time*, 19 April 1993, 41.

16. Barbier et al., "Parasitic Hazard with Sewage Sludge Applied to Land," *Applied and Environmental Microbiology* 56, no. 5 (May 1990): 1420-22.

17. Stanley Weinberger, *Parasites: An Epidemic in Disguise* (Larkspur, California: Healing Within Products, 1993).

18. Ann Louise Gittleman. *Guess What Came to Dinner: Parasites and Your Health* (Garden Park City, New York: Avery Publishers, 1993).

19. Ann Louise Gittleman, "Intestinal Integrity," *Health World* (November/December 1989): 13-16.

20. Raeburn.

Chapter Seven

1. Brian Inglis and Ruth West, *The Alternative Health Guide* (New York, New York: Alfred Knopf, 1983), 121.

2. Huang Ti, *Nei Ching So Ben: The Yellow Emperor's Classic of Internal Medicine* (Los Angeles, California: University of California Press, 1966).

3. I. G. Dox et al., *Harper Collins Illustrated Medical Dictionary* (New York, New York: Harper Perennial, 1993), 7.

4. Ibid., 334.

5. John N. Ott, *Health and Light: The Effects of Natural and Artificial Light on Man and Other Living Things* (Old Greenwich, Connecticut: Devin Adair, 1973).

6. S. S. Kim, "Acupuncture Works—Like a Computer!" *American Journal of Acupuncture* 14, no. 2 (April/June 1986): 159-60.

7. Academy of Traditional Chinese Medicine. *An Outline of Chinese Acupuncture* (1975; reprint, Monterey Park, California: Chan's Corporation Languages Press, 1979), 31-32.

8. Kim.

9. Paul Marcus, *Acupuncture—A Patient's Guide* (New York: Thorsons Publishers, 1985), 112, reviewed in American Journal of Acupuncture (April/June 1986): 187.

10. L. L. Sacks, "Drug Addiction, Alcoholism, Smoking and Obesity Treated by Auricular Staplepuncture," *American Journal of Acupuncture* 3, no. 2 (April/June 1975): 147-50.

11. R. M. Giller, "Auricular Acupuncture and Weight Reduction," *American Journal of Acupuncture* 3, no. 2 (April/June 1975): 151-53.

12. E. L. Sun, "Weight Reduction with Auricular Acupressure," *American Journal of Acupuncture* 7, no. 4 (October/December 1979): 311-15.

13. Xu Bin et al., "Weight Reduction Treated by Auricular Therapy," *Chinese Acupuncture and Moxibustion* 4, no. 5 (December 1984): 17-18 (In Chinese).

14. Y. M. Sin et al., "Effect of Electric Acupuncture Stimulation On Acute Inflammation," *American Journal of Acupuncture* 11, no. 4 (October/December 1983): 359-62.

15. Y. M. Sin, "Acupuncture and Inflammation," *International Journal of Chinese Medicine* 1, no. 1 (March 1984): 15-20.

16. Ibid.

17. J. Bossy, "Immune Systems, Defense Mechanisms and Acupuncture," *American Journal of Acupuncture* 18, no. 3 (1990): 219-32.

18. C. Schwartz, "Treatment of Systemic Lupus Erthematosus with Acupuncture, Chinese Herbs and Homeopathy in a Dog," *American Journal of Acupuncture* 18, no. 3 (1990): 247-49. 19. Misha Cohen, "Chinese Medicine in the Treatment of Chronic Immunodeficiency: Diagnosis and Treatment," *American Journal of Acupuncture* 18, no. 2 (1990): 111-22.

20. Peter V. Pugach, "The Influence of Acupuncture on the Structure of Immune Organs," *American Journal of Acupuncture* 21, no. 1 (1993): 59-62.

21. He Hon Lao, "Acupuncture Treatment of Mycosis Fungoides," *American Journal of Acupuncture* 16, no. 3 (July/September 1988): 221-24.

22. R. J. Marshall et al., "The Use of Alternative Therapies by New Zealand General Practitioners," *New Zealand Medical Journal* (1990): 103, 213-15, cited in *American Journal of Acupuncture* 18, no. 3 (1990): 291.

23. "Pharmacists' Perceptions of Alternative Health Approaches," *Journal of Clinical Pharmacy and Therapeutics* 15, no. 2 (1990): 141-46, cited in *American Journal of Acupuncture* 18, no. 3 (1990): 291.

24. K. Johansson et al., "Can Sensory Stimulation Improve the Functional Outcome in Stroke Patients?" *Neurology* 43 (November 1993): 2189-192.

Chapter Eight

1. Phil Gunby, "Fiber Catches Fancy of Nutrition Congress," *Journal of American Medical Association* 238, no. 16 (17 October 1977): 1715-16.

2. Bernard Jensen, *Tissue Cleansing Through Bowel Management* (Escondido, California: Bernard Jensen Publishing, 1981), 3.

3. Leo Galland, "Nutrition and Candidiasis," *Journal of Orthomolecular Psychiatry* 14, no. 1 (Fall 1985): 50-60.

4. Andrew Gutaulas, "Cleanse the Colon to Check Candida," *AT LAST NewsLink* 1, no. 2 (May 1990): 8-9.

5. Sharon Begley et al., "Beyond Vitamins," *Newsweek*, 25 April 1994, 45-49.

6. Dennis Nelson, *Food Combining Simplified* (Santa Cruz, California: D. Nelson Publishing, 1988), 13-16.

7. Begley.

8. Ibid.

9. Gloria Bucco, "Why are Americans Choosing Alternative Medicine?" *Delicious* (July/August 1993): 16-20.

10. Begley.

11. Keith Schneider, "Low Levels of Dioxin May Threaten Immune System," *New York Times*, cited in St. Paul Pioneer Press (11 May 1994): 1, 5.

12. M. M. Van Benschoten, "Toxic Residues in Common Foods," *American Journal of Acupuncture* 21, no. 2 (1993): 163-69.

13. Ruth Winter, MS, *A Consumer's Dictionary of Food Additives* (New York: Crown Trade Paperbacks, 1994), 319.

14. John Parks Trowbridge and Morton Walker, *The Yeast Connection* (New York, New York: Bantam Books, 1986), 361.

Chapter Nine

1. Michio Kuski, *Your Face Never Lies* (Wayne, New Jersey: Avery Publishing Group, 1983), 82.

2. Brian Inglis and Ruth West, "Iridology," in *Alternative Health Guide* (New York, New York: Knopf, 1983), 279.

3. Ralph Alan Dale, "The Micro-Acupuncture System," *American Journal of Acupuncture* (January/March 1976): 7-24 and (July/September 1976): 196-223.

4. Glenn J. Knox, "Colon Hydrotherapy and Enemas," *I-Act Quarterly* (International Association for Colon Therapy, Spring 1994): 16.

5. Tohru Tsukahza, "Fungicidal Action of Caprylic Acid for Candida Albicans," *Japanese Journal of Microbiology* 5, no. 4 (1961): 383-94.

6. Maurizio Trevisan et al., "Consumption of Olive Oil, Butter, and Vegetable Oils and Coronary Heart Disease Risk Factors," *Journal of the American Medical Association* 263, no. 5 (2 February 1990): 688-92.

7. Kerry Pechter, "The Amazing Benefits of the New Fiber Supplements," *Prevention* (October 1982): 28-29.

8. Ibid.

9. Jennifer Newman, "The Breakfast Drug," *American Health* (December 1989): 82-85.

10. Ibid.

11. Frederic Damru, "The Value of Bentonite for Diarrhea," *Medical Annals of the District of Columbia* 30, no. 6 (June 1961): 326-28.

12. Dalton Moore, "Candida Can Be Totally Destroyed," *Alive: Canadian Journal of Health and Nutrition* 112 (September 1991).

13. Ibid.

14. Ibid.

15. J. O. Hunter, "Food Allergy—Or Enteometabolic Disorder?" *Lancet* 338 (24 August 1991): 495-96, cited in *Clinical Pearls*, 190.

16. Moore.

17. Douglas Hunt. *No More Cravings* (New York, New York: Warner Books, 1987), 116.

Chapter Ten

1. James Balch and Phyllis Balch, *Prescription for Nutritional Healing* (Garden City Park, New York: Avery Publishing Group, 1990), 125.

2. Nafsika Georgopapadakou and Thomas Walsh, "Human Mycoses: Drugs and Targets for Emerging Pathogens," *Science* 264 (April 1994): 371.

3. M. M. Van Benschoten, "Management of Systemic Fungal Infections by Chinese Herbal Medicine," *American Journal of Acupuncture* 18, no. 3 (1990): 241-45.

4. Larry Wilson, Nutritional Balancing and Hair Mineral Analysis (Scottsdale, Arizona: L. D. Wilson Consultants, 1991), 140-41.

5. Van Benschoten.

6. Balch, 125.

7. Michael Weiner. *The People's Herbal* (New York, New York: Putnam Publishing Group, 1984), 183-90.

8. Van Benschoten.

9. Ibid.

10. John Parks Trowbridge and Morton Walker, *The Yeast Syndrome* (New York, New York: Bantam Books, 1986), 157.

11. Balch, 56.

12. Robert Rothenberg, *Medical Dictionary and Health Manual* (New York, New York: New American Library, 1988), 360.

13. Dian D. Buchman, *Medical Mysteries* (New York, New York: Scholastic, Press, 1992), 91.

14. Balch, 4.

15. Rothenberg, 360.

16. Shari Lieberman and Nancy Bruning, *The Real Vitamin and Mineral Book* (Garden City Park, New York: Avery Publishing Group, 1990), 66, 88.

17. Balch, 4.

18. Mark Bricklin, *Prevention's Giant Book of Health Facts* (Emmaus, PA: Rodale Press, 1991), 545.

19. David Larson, *Mayo Clinic Family Health Book* (New York, New York: William Morrow & Co., 1990), 363.

20. Lieberman, 56.

21. Wilson, 219-20.

22. Watson, 348.

23. Wilson 140.

24. Gary Young; "Together," *Young Living News and Information* (January 1994): 1.

25. Gary Young, "Essential Oils," (lecture, Minneapolis, MN, 12 April 1994).

26. Young, "Together," 1.

27. Ibid.

28. Balch, 323.

29. Nicholas Gonzalez, "No Toxicity with Coffee Enemas or Laetrile," *Townsend Letter for Doctors* (November 1988): 496, 497.

30. Van Benschoten.

31. Kasuga Yoshida et al., "Antifungal Activity of Ajoene Derived from Garlic," *Applied and Environmental Microbiology* 53, no. 3 (March 1987): 615-17.

32. Sharma G. Prasad, "Efficacy of Garlic Gallium Sativum Treatment Against Experimental Candidiasis in Chicks," *British Veterinarian Journal* 136, no. 5 (1980): 448-51.

33. Jane E. Brody, "After 4,000 Years Medical Science Considers Garlic," *New York Times*, 4 September 1990.

34. FC&A Staff, "Keep Your Brain Young—Walk," *New Natural Healing Encyclopedia* (Peachtree, Georgia: FC&A Publishing, 1990), 245.

35. Martha Slattery, David Jacobs, and Milton Nichaman, "Leisure Time Physical Activity and Coronary Heart Disease Death," *Circulation* 79, no. 2 (February 1989): 304-11.

36. Rothenberg, 241.

Chapter Twelve

1. Jeffrey Bland, "Candid Talk About Candida," *Delicious* (November/December 1988): 6-9.

2. James Balch and Phyllis Balch, "Simple Versus Complex Carbohydrates," *Prescription for Nutritional Healing* (Garden City Park, New York: Avery Publishing, 1990), 14, 15.

3. Michael Schmidt, Lendon Smith, and Keith Sehnert, *Beyond Antibiotics* (Berkeley, California: North Atlantic Books, 1993), 85.

4. A. Sanchez et al., "Role of Sugars in Human Neutorphilic Phagocytosis," *American Journal of Clinical Nutrition* 26 (1973), 180, cited in Michael Schmidt, Lendon Smith, and Keith Sehnert, *Beyond Antibiotics* (Berkeley, California: North Atlantic Books, 1993), 83-85.

5. Schmidt, 84.

6. Balch, 14, 15.

7. A. V. Constantini, "Dietary Choices Increase or Decrease the Mycotoxin Connection," Symposion fuer Umwelmedizin, Emstal, Germany, 25-27 September 1992.

8. John Trowbridge and Morton Walker, "The Yeast Control Diet," *The Yeast Syndrome* (New York, New York: Bantam Books, 1986), 187-227.

9. Douglas Hunt, *No More Cravings* (New York, New York: Warner Books, 1987), 142.

10. Linda Murray, "Creative Juicing," *Self*, May 1992, 125.

11. N. W. Walker, *Fresh Vegetable and Fruit Juices* (Prescott, Arizona: Norwalk Press, 1970), 10-11.

12. Stuart Berger, *Dr. Berger's Immune Power Diet* (New York, New York: New American Library, 1985), 60-61.

13. Ibid.

14. Crook, 202.

15. Trowbridge, 188.

16. Crook, 293-94.

17. Trowbridge, 188.

18. Andrew Wail, *Natural Health, Natural Medicine* (Boston, Massachusetts: Houghton Mifflin, 1990), 33.

19. Trowbridge, 212, 223.

20. Berger, 60-61.

21. Gail Nielsen, "NutraSweet," *Candida Research and Information Foundation Newsletter* 9 (March 1989): 35.

22. Edna Zeavin, "The Outlaw Herbal Sweetener," *East West* (February 1988): 28, 29.

23. Weil, 56-57.

24. Weil, 55.

Chapter Thirteen

1. Keith Sehnert, *Selfcare/Wellcare* (Minneapolis, Minnesota: Augsburg Publishing House, 1985), 120.

2. Y. M. Sin, "Effect of Electric Acupuncture Stimulation on Acute Inflammation," *American Journal of Acupuncture* 11, no. 4 (October/December 1983).

3. Y. M. Sin, "Acupuncture and Inflammation," *International Journal of Chinese Medicine* 1, no. 1 (March 1984): 15-20.

4. Sehnert.

5. S. Lovacky, et al., "Plasma Beta Endorphin and Serum Bombesin Levels During Acupuncture Treatment of Duodenal Cancer," *American Journal of Acupuncture* 18, no. 2 (1990): 105-10.

6. Michael Murray and Joseph Pizzorno, "Impaired Liver Function," in *Encyclopedia of Natural Medicine* (Rocklin, California: Prima Publishing, 1991), 185.

7. Rupert Beebe, *Candida Yeast Infection: The Silent Killer* (Vancouver, B.C. Canada: Healthology, 1988), 375.

Chapter Fourteen

1. Andrew Weil, *Natural Health, Natural Medicine* (Boston, Massachusetts: Houghton Mifflin, 1990), 236-237.

2. Weil, 239-40.

3. James Balch and Phyllis Balch, *Prescription for Nutritional Healing* (Garden City Park, New York: Avery Publishing, 1990), 40-41.

4. Michael Murray and Joseph Pizzorno, *An Encyclopedia of Natural Medicine* (Rocklin, California: Prima Publishing, 1991), 61-62.

5. Keith Sehnert, *Selfcare/Wellcare*, (Minneapolis, Minnesota: Augsburg Publishing House, 1985), 58-59.

6. Balch, 319.

7. Ross Trattler, *Better Health Through Natural Healing* (New York, New York: McGraw-Hill, 1985), 561.

8. John Trowbridge and Morton Walker, *The Yeast Syndrome*, (New York, New York: Bantam Books, 1986), 61-62.

9. Trattler, 243.

10. Trattler, 289.

11. Trattler, 292.

12. Trattler, 293.

13. Trattler, 439.

14. William G. Crook, *The Yeast Connection*, (Jackson, Tennessee: Professional Books, 1986), 316.

15. Crook, 150.

16. Crook, 146.

17. Crook, 151.

18. Lawrence Wilson, *Nutritional Balancing and Hair Mineral Analysis*, (Scottsdale, Arizona: L. D. Wilson Consultants, 1991), 115.

19. Marcia Starck, *The Complete Handbook of Natural Healing* (St. Paul, Minnesota: Llewellyn Publications, 1991), 203.

20. Starck 203-4.

21. Wilson, 266.

22. Ibid.

23. Wilson, 205-6.

24. Wilson, 207-8.